CW00409143

TRANS FAT

The Time Bomb in Your Food

How a killer ingredient in thousands of our daily food choices is increasing our risk of heart disease five-fold and saving the food industry millions of pounds.

MAGGIE STANFIELD

SOUVENIR PRESS

Copyright © 2008 by Maggie Stanfield

First published in 2008 by Souvenir Press Ltd
43 Great Russell Street, London WC1B 3PD

The right of Maggie Stanfield to be identified as the author
of this work has been asserted by her in accordance with
the Copyright, Designs and Patents Act, 1988

All rights reserved. No part of this publication may be reproduced,
stored in a retrieval system or transmitted, in any form or by any means,
electronic, mechanical, photocopying, or otherwise, without the prior
permission of the Copyright owner.

The Publisher makes no representation, express or implied,
with regard to the accuracy of the information contained in this
work, and legal responsibility or liability cannot be accepted by
the Author or the Publisher for any errors or omissions that
may be made or for any loss, damage, injury or problems
suffered or in any way arising from following the nutritional
advice offered in these pages.

ISBN 9780285638198

Typeset by M Rules

Printed and bound in Great Britain

CONTENTS

FOREWORD

We're bombarded daily with information about what we're eating, whether it's good or bad for us, if it causes allergies or cancer, hyperactivity or obesity. One day we hear that eating organic is ideal and a week later we're told that it is a good way to contract Avian Flu.

The confusion caused is music to the ears of the food manufacturers who know very well that we all tend to sigh and hope for the best. There are, after all, stringent EU regulations about the safety of our food, aren't there? Look at BSE and foot and mouth disease or Avian Flu. We've seen tens of thousands of animals destroyed just in case any one of them is infected. Surely we can trust the experts to ensure we are eating food that is safe?

Wrong! We are consuming damaging chemical and industrial products on a daily basis and we are not being given the information that would allow us to avoid them. We don't need them; they have no nutritional value; and we ought to get rid of them. They include some of the E-numbers that add colours, preservatives, emulsifiers and flavourings to our food and – most dangerous of all – they include trans fat.

There is a lot of confusion and a lack of consensus about the potential damage certain E-numbers can cause, yet although the actual numbers must be listed on the ingredients panels of food packaging, we get no indication of the associated risks. That's why this book contains a directory listing of all the main E-numbers in use in the UK, with the potential risks associated with each. Many E-numbers are perfectly safe, but you can make up your own mind about the suspect ones with the help of this directory. Anyone with young children, with a tendency to food allergies or stomach disorders should look closely at this guide. We have a generation of young children taking amphetamines like Ritalin when all that may be required is the removal of certain food additives.

Many families with children suffering from Attention Deficit Hyperactivity Disorder (ADHD) are already aware of the dangers of E102 Tartrazine, which is already banned in several countries. E110 is an azo yellow colourant associated with kidney tumours and is banned in most European countries, but it is still in use in the UK. Then there's the E210-E219 group of benzoates, preservatives made from toluene, which is a by-product of crude oil. Dr John Larsen, who heads the European Food Safety Authority's panel on additives, has said it would be 'prudent' to remove them from children's food. An extensive report published late in 2007 by a research team at the University of Southampton has warned that additives harm the 'psychological health' of children, holding back their progress at school and their ability to learn to read at a young age.[1]

We need to be far more watchful when it comes to what we eat because the food industry isn't going to tell us very much. What it does include in the ingredients panel won't detail the dangers. Inadequate labelling and miniscule lettering is a very efficient way of making sure we don't ask awkward questions that might threaten to cut into profit margins.

There is no confusion at all about trans fat. The evidence is overwhelming and well documented. Many of the foods we buy are loaded with it: confectionery, stock cubes, frozen meals, deep-fried foods, takeaway snacks, biscuits, pastries, desserts, even vitamin capsules and 'wholesome' cereal bars, to name just a handful.

Most people have never even heard of trans fat, have no idea what it is, and so see no reason to avoid it, and why should they?

1 'Food additives and hyperactive behaviour in 3 and 8/9 year old children in the community' Jim Stevenson et al, University of Southampton Schools of Psychology and Medicine, September 2007

You won't find it listed in the ingredients or for sale on the super-market shelves. You won't see it mentioned in the nutrition panel or much discussed in articles about nutrition and diet. It is much easier for the food manufacturers: if we don't know, we won't complain.

Trans fat is basically hydrogenated vegetable oil. It is the industrial processing of the oil, not the oil itself that creates the killer trans fat. Make no mistake; trans fat is lethal. It contributes to obesity, Type II diabetes, allergies, and most of all, heart disease. Just one doughnut a day that contains trans fats could be increasing your risk of heart disease five-fold.

That's why this book is so necessary. It gives you the information you need so that you are equipped to make intelligent, informed choices for you and your family.

Eight of the big UK supermarket multiples announced in January 2007 that they would voluntarily remove hydrogenated vegetable oils (HVOs) from their own-brand products. Asda, Boots, Co-Op, Iceland, Marks & Spencer, Sainsbury's, Tesco and Waitrose promised it would be done by the end of 2007, but by the end of the year, it is still easy to find plenty of these products on the shelves.

Sainsbury's told us in July 2007 that 'we have removed all hydrogenated vegetable oils from our entire range of own label foods and drinks', yet we were still able to find HVOs in the ingredients lists of Sainsbury-branded foods. Asda, too, had a raft of own-brand products featuring the deadly ingredient in November and December 2007.

Stephen Crabb MP, Chair of the All-Party Parliamentary Retail Industry Group, tabled a rather premature Early Day Motion on 30 January 2007 which stated: 'This House congratu-lates Asda, Boots, Co-Op, Iceland, Marks & Spencer, Sainsbury, Tesco and Waitrose for removing industrially created trans fats from their own brand lines; recognises that this move will help UK consumers choose a healthy, balanced diet; is encouraged to see UK retailers taking such significant steps to help reduce the risk of coronary heart disease in the UK; is proud that British retailers are leading the way in Europe by making such a com-mitment to the EU Platform on diet, physical activity and health;

and encourages the European food industry to follow this excellent example'.

While the big supermarkets account for just over half of our food sales (56 per cent), their own brand products are relatively small in number. It is the products they buy in from other manufacturers that largely fill our shopping baskets. These producers have made no commitment at all to withdrawing trans fats.

If we ate nothing but decent, honest food, prepared and cooked in our own homes, we would all be a lot healthier. However, very few of us never eat processed food, ready meals, takeaway foods, or in-store bakery cakes and pastries. Even the healthiest of us eat these products now and then. Nearly two out of three of people in the UK will be overweight by 2050, according to the Minister for Health.

In Denmark, the government decided that the health of their people was more important than the profits of Danish food manufacturers. The country banned the use of hydrogenated vegetable oil in 2003, and within three years had seen deaths from heart disease drop by over 20 per cent. The professor and nutritional expert who led the drive, Dr Steen Stender, said he didn't see why anyone should have to understand the complicated chemistry or even be familiar with the terms. It is down to governments to act on behalf of people. He believes the whole of the EU should do the same.

We could be killing 30,000 people a year with trans fats in the UK alone. Isn't it time to ban them once and for all?

ACKNOWLEDGEMENTS

A wealth of experts were supportive in bringing this book to fruition. I would especially like to thank Professor Steen Stender, Chairman of the Danish Nutrition Council, who drove forward that country's decision to ban the use of hydrogenated vegetable oil. I would also like to thank Wageningen University, Netherlands, for granting permission to use some of its Food Microbiology Group information on E-numbers. Oliver Tickell, the founder of www.tfx.org.uk, provided useful insights, and Alex Renton's *Guardian* feature is one of the best explanations of the subject that I have seen. I would also like to thank Ernest Hecht, my publisher, for his ongoing support and guidance and Becky Alexander for her perceptive editing.

CHAPTER 1

THE HIDDEN KILLER

There is a hidden killer ingredient in many of the foods that you and your family are eating. Unless you are living on a 100 per cent organic diet, you are almost certainly consuming it daily. If you have children, they will be victims too. Vegetarians and vegans are not exempt. If you follow an Atkins, wheat-free, dairy free or food-combining diet, you are at risk too. Any time you buy a takeaway or eat a Danish pastry from a supermarket bakery, you will almost certainly be getting a share of this product.

Although there have been some warnings about it, you may well be one of millions who have never heard of it or, if you have heard it mentioned, have no idea what it actually is. You can't see it, you won't find it as a product on a supermarket shelf, it isn't listed on the ingredients labels and even in the catering industry, it hides under different names. But it is killing us as surely and definitively as an outbreak of E-coli.

So what is it, this mysterious and threatening hidden ingredient that we are all innocently consuming? Trans fats. To give them their full title – triglycerides of fatty acids (TFAs), also known as trans isomer fatty acids.

Trans fats are unsaturated fatty acids created during the full or partial hydrogenation of vegetable oil (HVO or PHVO). During the industrial process that converts liquid vegetable oil into solid or semi-solid fat by boiling it to more than 260 degrees centigrade, these 'rogue' fat molecules are produced. Manufacturers use the fat to give texture (or 'mouth-feel') to food, and to help preserve it. In the UK, it is often used as a cheap replacement for butter in bakery goods.

For the sake of convenience, we refer throughout this book to trans fats and HVOs as mutually exchangeable terms because there is no such thing as an HVO that does not contain trans fat.

It is important to emphasis that while trans fats are more dangerous than saturated fats, too many saturated fats are not the answer either! We need to find healthy alternatives. The Danish Nutrition Council's report on trans fats, which led to that country's banning of industrially produced HVOs, points out that: 'Compared with saturated fat, the studies indicate that, gram for gram, industrially produced trans fatty acids increase the risk of heart disease considerably more (tenfold)'.[1]

The invention of trans fats

Back in 1903, an American chemist called Wilhelm Normann worked out that by boiling cottonseed oil to temperatures of more than 260°C, it would solidify. He saw that he could produce a cheap replacement for the animal-based tallow then used to make candles. As a result of his initial work, we've been spreading candle wax on our toast in the guise of margarine for the last 75 years or so.

It was the multi-national corporation, Proctor & Gamble, who bought the rights to Mr Normann's patent in 1909. Within a couple of years, the company was marketing the first hydrogenated shortening. Up until then, every housewife and kitchen-maid baked the family's food using entirely natural ingredients such as butter and lard. Certainly, the quotient of what we are now familiar with as saturated fat in most diets was high, but there were proportionately fewer heart attacks in the 1900s than now.

A wonder food

The American product that Proctor & Gamble launched was called *Crisco* and it was a huge success. A cookbook of *Crisco*

---

1 The influence of trans fatty acids on health, Fourth Edition, Danish Nutrition Council, Steen Stender et al

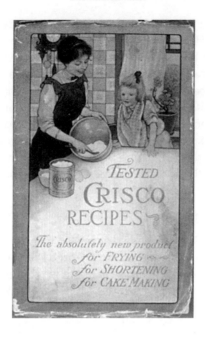

recipes was produced in 1912. A whole series followed, actively promoting the value of this magical product. There were cookbooks for the general public and ones specifically written for Japanese, Jewish or Philippine households. Titles included: *A Cookery Course in 13 Chapters; 24 Pies Men Like;* and *Crisco Recipes for the Jewish Housewife.* That *Crisco* contained no animal fat made it ideal for vegetarian, Kosher and Halal households.

The rationing and food shortages that hit kitchens during two World Wars helped *Crisco* grow in popularity. By 1945, *Crisco* was selling around the world, under various different brand names. You wouldn't find a shop, cáfé, hospital, railway dining car, or a fish and chip shop without it. Everyone assumed it was a good product because it was made from vegetable oil.

The raw ingredient then was cottonseed oil, but these days it is more usually soybean oil. It was made into semi-solid products that were easy to rub in with flour and produced a rich, melt-in-the-mouth flavour and texture at a far lower price than butter.

The UK market followed with well-known products like Trex, Echo, Spry, Stork, Cookeen and Pura made in the same way.

Housewives loved these products. They were cheap, easy to work with, had a long shelf-life and didn't impart any unwanted flavours into the end product. It looked like an ideal substitute for butter. It was promoted as pure as the driven snow, the whiteness of the bleached product being equated with naturalness. It could be stored on the kitchen shelf easily and didn't even need to be refrigerated (at a time when few households owned a refrigerator, shelf life was an important attribute).

The legacy today

Only in the last 15 years have we realised that the hydrogenation process produces this damaging by-product: trans fatty acids. When the raw vegetable oil is heated to great intensity, the molecules are shaken up so much that the atomic structure of the oil is actually altered.

Many deep-fried foods, whether from up-market restaurants, câfés, or takeaway shops will have been cooked in these blocks of fat. They are used because they melt down easily, can be heated to high temperatures, and can be re-used many times.

Many bakery goods, such as cakes, biscuits and snack bars contain trans fats. The food industry experts talk about HVOs as having 'good mouth feel'. You can even manufacture 'luxury mouth feel' by hydrogenating certain oils so that they literally 'melt in the mouth' like butter, hence their popularity with bakery manufacturers. Even some so-called 'healthy' energy cereal bars contain trans fats, while at the same time proclaiming their wholesomeness and 'natural' ingredients.

Some people believe that trans fats are used only in the fast food industry. This simply isn't true, although takeaway foods have high levels of trans fat, sometimes as much as 40 per cent of their overall fat content. Avoiding traditional 'junk food' outlets and products will not protect you from this attacker.

Foods that contain these chemically created trans fats may have nearly half their fat content in this form. Baking fats of the HVO kind will have around a third of their fat content as trans fats while the animal or natural forms contain perhaps two or three per cent of their total fat as trans fats. Some margarines can contain up to 15 per cent trans fat by weight.

Trans fat levels can be measured in a laboratory. The techniques include chromatography, where the layers of different fats are separated out. Spectroscopy can also be used, but when it comes to working it out for ourselves, we are helpless.

Hydrogenated fats will almost certainly be lurking in a range of foods in your kitchen cupboard today. Even luxury food items like chocolate truffles and soft caramels regularly contain trans fats. We, unknowingly, eat a product used to make candles, although it won't be describing itself as candle wax. Many of us consume it even when eating out in expensive restaurants. The idea of a romantic 'candlelit dinner' begins to take on a whole new meaning!

Banish trans fats forever!

This book gives you all the information you need to get trans fats out of your kitchen and out of your life. The knowledge here is your key to identifying an ingredient you may well have been unaware even existed. Your cells, currently absorbing trans fat and increasingly confused by it, will be able to revert to their normal relationship with the vital omega-3 fats they need for renewal. You can halt the downward slide towards heart disease.

For anyone with children, this information is even more essential. If our diet continues to slide rapidly downhill, it is our children who will suffer most of all. As parents, many of us are going to find that we outlive them because we had a healthier childhood diet. This is in spite of our relative prosperity.

The heart disease time-bomb

Man-made trans fats are potentially lethal. One clinical health study found that increasing trans fat intake even in very small amounts could raise the risk of heart disease by a factor of ten or twelve.[2]

2 Trans Fatty Acids and Cardiovascular Disease, Mozaffarian, Willett et al, New England Journal of Medicine April 2006

The study found:

'On a per-calorie basis, trans fats appear to increase the risk of CHD (Coronary Heart Disease) more than any other macronutrient, conferring a substantially increased risk at low levels of consumption (1 to 3 percent of total energy intake). In a meta-analysis of four prospective cohort studies involving nearly 140,000 subjects, including updated analyses from the two largest studies, a 2 per cent increase in energy intake from trans fatty acids was associated with a 23 percent increase in the incidence of CHD.'

We need a ban in the UK

There is no safe level of trans fat intake. Hydrogenated vegetable oil, in all of its guises, has to go – and go completely from the human diet. Its use is already banned in Denmark. The rest of the world needs to follow suit.

In the United States, experts believe that up to 100,000 lives a year could be saved if HVOs and PHVOs were removed completely from the American diet. Here in the UK, if we translate that to our population figures, we could be talking about saving *30,000 lives a year* with a ban on trans fats.

Know your fats!

There has been so much information and advice about fats over the last 20 years or so that many people are thoroughly confused about 'good' and 'bad' fats. There is no real consensus on how much fat is healthy in our diet, nor really on where it should come from.

Some fats are good for us. In fact, some are essential for good health, so it is important to understand the distinction between trans fatty acids and good fats. They should never be confused.

Fats and oils are made mostly of fatty acids. All fatty acids are chains of carbon atoms with hydrogen atoms attached to the carbon atoms. A saturated fatty acid has the maximum possible number of hydrogen atoms attached to every carbon atom. This is why it is described as 'saturated' with hydrogen atoms. The chemical and physical properties of a fat are determined by the relative amounts of the various fatty acids it contains.

Generally, the higher the saturated fatty acid content, the harder the fat will be at room temperature; the more unsaturated fatty acids it contains, the more oil-like it will be. All fats contain a mixture of different fatty acids.

The knowledge gap

Some 97 per cent of adults in the UK are thoroughly confused about good and bad fats, what fats are found in what foods, which ones are good to eat and which not to eat, whether we really need fat at all and if so in what form.

The Fat Panel (www.thefatpanel.org.uk) is an independent UK-based group that has recently (2007) been established to provide objective information about the role and benefits of oils and fats and what we need to do to get the right dietary balance. It questioned 551 adults about fats. Around half of the respondents did not realise that dietary fat is important for:

- Tissue repair
- Healthy skin
- Protecting the internal organs
- Transporting vitamins around the body
- Hormone metabolism

And almost half of respondents did not know that cutting saturated fat intake would reduce the risk of developing cardiovascular disease, Type II diabetes and some cancers. But more than one in five (22 per cent) think that cutting down the saturated fat in their diet will improve their love lives.

Most of those surveyed were able to identify lard, butter, pastry and meat products as being high in saturated fats (around 90 per cent knew this). Less than half of those questioned recognised that saturated fats were very bad for health and more than 10 per cent thought these kinds of fat were good for us.

On trans fats, 80 per cent of those surveyed had no idea that these fats were dangerous and nearly a fifth (16 per cent) actually thought they were good for us. Nearly a quarter of the survey thought the essential omega-3 trans fatty acids were bad for us and a third thought monounsaturated fats were bad news.

The low-down on the good, bad and the ugly

It is important that we understand enough about the different fat groups to be able to select foods that will not expose us to the elevated heart disease risks associated with *trans* and saturated fats. There are four major types of fats in the foods we eat:

- **Saturated fatty acids or saturated fats** The term 'saturated' means that these fats have all the hydrogen the carbon atoms can hold. Traditionally, this is the fat group we have been told to avoid most of all but nutritionists are now recognising that limited amounts of saturated fat are actually less damaging than trans fats. Saturated fats are usually solid at room temperature, and they are more stable which means that they do not combine readily with oxygen and turn rancid. The most familiar saturated fat in the British diet is butter but hard cheese also has high levels. Curd or cottage cheese has a low fat content. Saturated fats in the diet may raise blood cholesterol, which can increase the risk of coronary heart disease and stroke. Saturated fatty acids are found in foods from animals (meat, dripping and whole-milk dairy products), coconut, palm and palm kernel oils, and cocoa butter.
- **Monounsaturated fatty acids** These fatty acids are found in canola, olive and peanut oils, avocados, and nuts. These oils are liquid at room temperature but start to solidify when chilled. For example, salad dressing containing olive oil turns cloudy when refrigerated but is clear at room temperature. Monounsaturated fatty acids can help decrease LDL or 'bad' cholesterol and may contribute to protecting heart health.

- **Polyunsaturated fatty acids** Liquid at room temperature and when chilled. They do not last as long in the deep fryer. Polyunsaturated fatty acids can help lower LDL cholesterol when substituted for saturated fats in the diet. Polyunsaturated fatty acids are found in safflower, sesame, sunflower, corn and soybean oils, fatty fish (salmon, mackerel, smelt, herring and trout), walnuts and seeds.
- **Trans fatty acids (trans fats)** A specific type of fat formed when liquid oils are made into solid fats like shortening and hard or 'stick' margarine in the 'partial hydrogenation' process. Trans fats are also found naturally in small amounts in certain foods (for example, dairy products, beef and lamb). Trans fats raise LDL cholesterol levels and lower the 'good' HDL cholesterol which we require for cell repair. Trans fats are found in foods made with, or fried in, partially and fully hydrogenated oils.

The essential building blocks

Essential fatty acids (EFAs) are the building blocks of fats. They are important within human chemistry because they occupy every cell membrane, most of our major organs and are crucial to our immune system function. Don't get confused between trans fatty acids (TFA) and essential fatty acids. Though the tags sound similar, these are very different components in our biology. Naturally occurring essential fatty acids have an electrical weight that changes the fluidity of cell membranes. This is important to how our immune cells develop.

When oils are hydrogenated, the electrical weight is changed. This in turn alters the fluidity of the cell membrane, making it stiffen up. When we consume trans fats, our bodies are unable to synthesize them properly, and starts to form abnormal cells.

We cannot produce our own EFAs so we need to get them from fish and vegetable oils in the correct ratios. There are three vital essential fatty acids: linoleic omega-6 type; linoleic acid N omega-4 type; and alpha-linolenic N, the omega-3 type.

It is time to set the record straight in an easy to understand way. We do *need* certain fats (especially omega-3 fatty acids which our bodies can't produce for themselves and which are vital for cell replenishment) and a totally fat-free diet would be very damaging to our health and cell structure. What we certainly do *not* need is artificially manufactured fats that distort nature.

We know that as a nation we consume too much saturated fat, but the UK Government Food Standards Agency is only now consulting towards the production of a draft saturated fat and energy intake programme. Its position at the moment is:

'Current population average intakes of saturated fat exceed public health recommendations and the rising levels of obesity indicate that energy (calorie) intakes currently exceed energy requirements. Both these conditions raise serious health concerns, particularly in relation to cardiovascular disease, some cancers and Type 2 diabetes.

The Agency is currently consulting on its draft saturated fat and energy intake programme, which aims to reduce saturated fat intakes and contribute to helping consumers achieve and maintain energy balance.'

The American Department of Agriculture (which deals with the national interest in food and nutrition) suggests that a fat intake of more than 35 per cent of calories will make it difficult to avoid putting on excess weight while a low intake of less than 20 per cent of calories increases the risk of being deficient in vitamin E and the essential fatty acids. Too little of the right fats can also distort the balance between 'good' and 'bad' cholesterol.

How much fat should you eat?

The American Department of Agriculture provides the following key recommendations:

- Consume less than 10 per cent of your daily calories from saturated fatty acids and less than 300 mg/day of cholesterol, and keep *trans* fatty acid consumption as low as possible.
- Keep your total fat intake between 20 to 35 percent of your daily calories, with most fats coming from sources of polyunsaturated and monounsaturated fatty acids, such as fish, nuts, and vegetable oils.
- When selecting and preparing meat, poultry, dry beans and milk or milk products, make choices that are lean, low-fat, or fat-free.
- Limit intake of fats and oils high in saturated and/or *trans* fatty acids, and choose products low in such fats and oils.[3]

Children need fat

Young children (aged between two and three years old) need slightly higher levels of fat intake – up to 35 per cent of their diet. Children from the ages of four to 18 should keep fat intake between 25 and 35 per cent of total calories consumed. Most of the fat sources should be polyunsaturated and monounsaturated fatty acids, such as fish, nuts and vegetable oils.

Cutting out trans fats could do as much to improve our health as stopping smoking.

Is it on the label?

How do you choose what to buy from the array of margarines and various butter and baking alternatives? The confusing marketing

---

3 United States Department of Agriculture Dietary Guidelines for Americans 2005

messages make choosing very difficult. Things are, indeed, not always what they seem. Partially hydrogenated vegetable oil has various disguises: shortening, margarine, partially hydrogenated soybean or cottonseed oil. On the nutrition panel, trans fats are often buried within the unsaturated fats measure, even though our bodies are quite unable to process trans fats as unsaturates.

Since January 2006, America has stipulated that trans fat content must be included on every nutrition label. However, we in the UK are not being given the same information. Although legally, manufacturers must list HVOs in the ingredients, this information is often in such a small font size and buried under a paper fold that it would take a veritable Sherlock Holmes with a magnifying glass to tease it out. Besides, the depressing reality is that legal requirements are probably not always met by food preparers and manufacturers.

One example of the fact that you can't always believe what you read is that a recent survey of beef mince revealed that 'extra lean' mince could contain as much or more fat than the ordinary 'standard' labelled product. The UK Food Standards Agency looked at 561 samples of fresh and frozen minced beef and found that:

- The amount of fat in standard beef mince ranged from 1.9g to 32.3g per 100g
- Several samples of 'extra' or 'super' lean mince actually had higher fat contents than some 'lean' mince
- 55 of the 308 samples giving nutrition information on the label contained more fat than the label claimed.

The chemistry of trans fats

If you are not interested in the chemistry of trans fats, you can skip this section.

Not everyone will want to understand the complexities of how trans fats are produced. For those of you who are interested in the chemistry, here is the background:

Fats are large E-shaped molecules that support three fatty acids on a spine. Fatty acid molecules have a spine with carbon atoms surrounded by hydrogen atoms. The way fats are categorised as saturated or unsaturated refers to the number of hydrogen atoms in the acid. If the molecule contains the maximum possible number, then it is saturated. Otherwise, it is unsaturated.

In saturated fatty acids, each carbon atom is connected to its two neighbour carbon atoms as well as two hydrogen atoms. In unsaturated fatty acids, the carbon atoms without hydrogen atoms are joined by double bonds rather than single ones, so each carbon atom still has four bonds.

Hydrogenation of an unsaturated fatty acid means bubbling in hydrogen atoms at a high temperature in the presence of a metal catalyst like nickel or another aluminium alloy.

What happens then is that the carbon atoms take on new hydrogen partners so as to maintain their four bonds per carbon atom and the double bonds change to single ones. Partial hydrogenation reconfigures most of the double bonds that do not become chemically saturated, twisting them so that the hydrogen atoms end up on different sides of the chain. It is this configuration that gives rise to the label *trans*, which means 'across' in Latin.

The normal *cis* configuration has been flipped over. The molecules have been *trans*-formed. The unsaturated fat starts to look and behave like a saturated one.

Industrial hydrogenation is mostly of the partial type because it is at this stage of the process that a malleable fat, solid at room temperature, is produced. It will melt as it is baked or consumed. Fully hydrogenated fat is more the texture of the candle wax, as Wilhelm Normann intended.

Natural trans fats

You will sometimes come across references to 'natural' trans fats. *Trans*-double bonds can occur in nature as the result of fermentation in grazing animals, so lamb, beef and dairy products do contain some trans fats. These quantities are very small and are not the result of an industrial process. Natural trans fats don't harm us and don't confuse our digestive systems. Broadly, the animal sources may have 0.5 to 2.5 per cent of the fat content as *trans* molecules while a bucket of Kentucky-style deep fried chicken might give you 40 per cent.

Diagram of the molecular structure of different fatty acids

Saturated fat	*Cis*-unsaturated fatty acid	*Trans*-unsaturated fatty acid
Saturated carbon atoms (each with two hydrogen molecules) joined by a single bond	Unsaturated carbon atoms (each with one hydrogen molecule) joined by a double bond. *Cis*-configuration.	Unsaturated carbon atoms (each with one hydrogen molecule) joined by a double bond and flipped over into the *Trans*-configuration.

CHAPTER 2

THE FOOD LABEL CONTROVERSY

Food labelling is controversial. One of the arguments Danish nutritionists gave in 1995 in favour of banning trans fats was that people don't read labels. On the other hand, clearer labelling would at least offer consumers a level of choice that they do not currently have.

In the United States, the Federal Drug Administration has now forced manufacturers to list trans fats and some states have gone further. The Mayor of New York has banned restaurants from using hydrogenated vegetable oils. If consumers with purchasing power insist on change and refuse to buy foods that contain trans fats, then the industry will have to respond. In the meantime, there is a certain amount of detective work involved.

The most effective approach to avoiding trans fats until labelling is improved is three-pronged:

1: Look for partially hydrogenated-anything on the ingredients list

If hydrogenation is mentioned at all, put it back on the shelf or if you are feeling in a campaigning spirit, take the product to the customer services desk and complain. If enough people do that, hydrogenated vegetable oils will vanish faster than melting butter. Some HVOs masquerade under various names, however, but this exclusion zone will cut out most offenders.

2: Train your own 'mouth feel'

This isn't as mysterious as it sounds. If the product is moist, a little chewy and tends to melt pleasingly in the mouth, it may well contain trans fats. Think of all those commercially baked cakes with coloured icing; moist, glazed Danish pastries; chewy chocolate chip cookies; doughnuts and moist coffee shop muffins. Other culprits include the glazed pastry you get on takeaway sausage rolls, Cornish pasties, pork pies and cheese filo pastry wraps. Many of these products are loaded with trans fats. You can quickly develop a seventh sense for the kinds of products likely to contain trans fats.

3: Ask questions

If you want to buy these products, and the label is not helpful, or is non-existent, ask the manager or person selling the food whether hydrogenated vegetable oils are used. Don't take 'I don't know' for an answer. If the local manager doesn't know, then find out where you can ask more questions. Someone, somewhere knows whether that company is using HVOs in its product range.

The in-store bakery scandal

Since the 1970s, most of the prepared, pre-packaged meals and snacks we purchase from supermarkets, takeaways, high street bakeries and coffee shops, have contained trans fats. Much of the time, even if we were being enthusiastic food detectives, we could not have known, because so many of these products are sold without any ingredients information. No law exists in the UK that forces manufacturers or retailers to provide this information about food produced in-store.

While researching this book, checks were made on a range of in-store bakeries at various supermarkets. In spite of Sainsbury's advertisement that 'information about allergens and ingredients is available from a member of the bakery team,' we found this not to be the case. At one branch, we were informed that Sainsbury's did not produce the in-store bakery products, that the cookies 'arrive in boxes' and that their ingredients were not known or available to either staff or customers. On none of our checks did the bakery team know where or how to find ingredient information.

Eight supermarket chains: Asda, Boots, Co-Op, Iceland, Marks & Spencer, Sainsbury, Tesco and Waitrose, have committed to removing trans fats from their own-brand produce by January 2008. However, most of the products we buy from supermarkets are made by external suppliers. The retailers, for all their purchasing power, will have to pressurise suppliers into producing trans fat-free goods.

Furthermore, things are not always quite what the Public Relations staff promise. In July 2007, a quick trip around one Sainsbury's branch in Edinburgh turned up a number of 'own brand' items which included hydrogenated vegetable oil in the ingredients listing. This included Sainsbury's Crumble Topping and Sainsbury's (frozen) Cod in Parsley Sauce. This, in spite of the public statement that no HVOs would be used in any Sainsbury's own brand product after December 2006.

Asda was still selling own-brand products containing HVOs in November 2007; with minimal effort, we found at least eight such products in one local branch.

Marks & Spencer has delivered. The company has now removed *all* HVOs from *all* its products. Since Autumn 2006, in advance of its January 2007 deadline, none of the food products on sale nationwide has contained any trans fats and that includes the in-store bakery products. Some information about ingredients is available from the bakery counter although this can be a little hit and miss around different branches. The corporate press office is a reliable and helpful source of precise information, including ingredients in specific products. Our detectives were unable to find any products in Marks & Spencer that contained hydrogenated vegetable oils.

Waitrose, too, has now removed trans fats from its own-brand produce but of course, it carries a great many lines that are not of its own manufacture. Its press office issued the statement that: 'All Waitrose own-label products are free from Hydrogenated Vegetable Oils (an ingredient linked to the presence of trans fats). This has been the case since the end of 2006'.

Tesco offered no information at its in-store bakery counter, but referred us to the corporate press office. It advised that: 'Tesco is committed to removing trans fats from its own-brand ranges'.

The press office did not respond to requests for specific information about in-store bakery products or about its time strategy in
spite of several invitations.

Are trans fats lurking in your food?

Legally speaking, manufacturers in the UK must list any
HVOs they use in the *ingredients* list on their products.
However, there is at least anecdotal evidence that not all
manufacturers have complied fully with this
requirement. To add to the confusion, the ingredient can
be described in a range of ways, making it difficult for a
shopper to find. To check if the food you pick up
contains trans fats, look for any of the following:

>   Partially hydrogenated fat
>   Hydrogenated vegetable oil
>   Partially hydrogenated vegetable oil
>   Hydrogenated vegetable fat
>   Vegetable fat partially hydrogenated
>   Vegetable oil and fat, partially hydrogenated
>   Vegetable fat and hydrogenated vegetable oil
>   Partially hydrogenated vegetable and animal fats
>   Mono- or di-glycerides of fatty acids
>   Vegetable shortening.
>   Vegetable suet crust

Understanding the labels

All packaged food in the UK lists the ingredients. Some products
also carry a *nutrition* panel. However, these panels vary from supermarket to supermarket, making it difficult to discern what the
information means, or to compare similar products from different
outlets. In the UK, what goes on the nutrition label is up to the food
manufacturer or retailer. You rarely find any mention of trans fats,
unless a specific nutrition claim such as 'low in trans fats' is made.
Most decide to include some information, but with mixed results.

The Tesco nutrition panel, for example, looks like this:

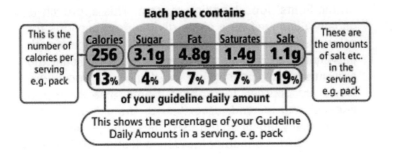

The information is confusing. Does this sandwich contain 4.8 grams of fat, or a total of 6.2 grams of fat (fat plus saturates)? What type of fat is the 4.8 grams? Poly- or monounsaturates? Are they animal or vegetable fats? Is there any trans fat? There is no way of telling from the information provided here.

This lack of consistency causes frustration and confusion for shoppers. The nutrition labels on, for example, three different makes of frozen lasagne, may not offer comparable information, so assessing which product offers the best nutrition and the least in terms of undesirable additives will be difficult, if not impossible.

The Food Standards Agency approach, championed by its chairwoman, Dame Deirdre Hutton CBE, has already met with resistance from a substantial group of retailers and manufacturers, including Tesco, Nestle, Unilever, Kellogg's, Cadbury Schweppes, Coca-Cola, Danone, Masterfoods and PepsiCo who have decided to take a different route with the Guideline Daily Amounts system. As a result, it is very difficult to make comparisons between products from different manufacturers displaying different systems. A review of an EU directive that governs the content and format of nutrition labels is under way, and may bring about change in the current regulations.

Red for danger, green for go

The UK Food Standards Agency recently introduced the 'traffic lights' food labelling system. This approach is usually displayed as a circle divided into sections for calories, fat, saturated fat, salt and total sugars with each coloured in green, amber or red to indicate the amounts of each per serving and depicting in red where levels are deemed to be high. Sometimes there is a linear listing instead, according to the colour danger levels. Many labels do not use this system at all.

The FSA's consumer guidance leaflet (which can be downloaded from: www.food.gov.uk) sets out the approach like this:

If you want to eat a healthy diet, one of the key things you can do is try to cut down on fat (especially saturated fat), salt and added sugars. When you are checking food labels to choose which products to buy, traffic light colours can help you make that choice quickly and easily.

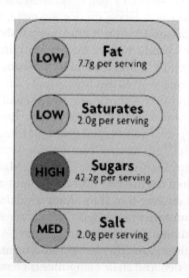

What the colours mean

Green means the food is low in fats, salt and/or sugar. The more green lights, the healthier the choice.

Amber means the food has a medium amount of fats, salt and/or sugar, so this is an OK choice most of the time, but you might want to go for a green option instead.

Red means the food is high in something we should be trying to cut down on. It's fine to have the food occasionally, or as a treat, but try to keep an eye on how often you choose these foods, or try eating them in smaller amounts.

Many foods with traffic light colours will have a mixture of greens, ambers and reds. So, when you're choosing between similar products, try to go for products with more greens and ambers, and fewer reds, to make the healthier choice.

Check it out

Some products you might have thought were healthy choices could qualify for red lights. Try comparing the saturated fat, sugar and salt levels of your favourite breakfast cereals with those that qualify for a full set of green lights.

A label conundrum

In 2006, a team of Oxford University scientists argued in the British Medical Journal that the UK should follow the American route, and start labelling trans fats alongside saturated, unsaturated and monounsaturated fats and cholesterol, so that consumers can make a more informed choice.

Even that logical way forward is not straightforward. The butter substitute, Benecol, claims to reduce cholesterol, yet it contained hydrogenated vegetable oil until very recently. The product has been reformulated now and contains no hydro-genated oil. The company was not lying, because the 'no trans fatty acids' claim complies with the US Drugs Administration regulations. It allows a company to make this claim providing the product contains no more than 0.5 grams of trans fats per serving. American dietary guidelines advise keeping trans fat intake under one gram a day.

However, Benecol advises users to 'spread it liberally at least three times a day'. It would, therefore, have been unexceptional to find an adult taking in two or three grams of trans fat a day while believing him or herself to be eating healthily.

How you can avoid trans fats

1. Don't eat products that have the words 'partially hydrogenated', 'hydrogenated vegetable oil', 'HVO', or 'shortening' in the ingredients list.
2. Be suspicious of labels that say 'no trans fats'. In some countries, amounts of less than 0.5 grams per serving (for example, the US) are considered 'none', but four cookies, each with 0.4 grams, would provide 1.6 grams of trans fat.
3. Although in the UK HVOs must, legally, be listed in the ingredients, this won't be true of products manufactured and purchased in many other countries.
4. When it comes to unlabelled and takeaway foods, be suspicious and ask questions. If we all keep asking 'does your food contain trans fats?' then the pressure will force manufacturers to seek alternatives. Non-packaged food is the greatest culprit.
5. In restaurants, câfés and pubs, ask what fats are used for frying, baking or in salad dressings. If you are told 'we use vegetable oil', ask if it is hydrogenated.
6. Lunchtime takeaway shops are probably among the most culpable when it comes to clogging up our arteries. You should especially avoid pasties, sausage rolls, pies, pastries, scones and cakes.
7. Monitor what your children are eating. Many branded confectionery bars, sweets, ice cream, popcorn and many

other products aimed specifically at children contain trans fats. If children are eating lunch at school, then ask about the use of trans fats in the school canteen.

Make a healthy choice

Medical research indicates that trans fats are far worse for health than the saturated fats that doctors tell us to avoid: trans fats raise LDL or 'bad cholesterol', while lowering HDL or 'good cholesterol'. They help gum up our arteries with fatty deposits. They have been identified as a significant cause of cardiovascular disease.

We need to equip ourselves with information to make choices that will not damage our long-term health. We need to demand that the food we buy declares its content in a clear, easy to understand way.

Better still, we need to be able to trust that the food choices we make do not contain hidden ingredients that will be damaging to us.

Why should we be forced to eat candle wax?

CHAPTER 3

HEALTH HAZARDS

As the heart disease epidemic scales ever greater heights, we need to ask ourselves what we can do to avoid being another statistic. We have more public information available than ever before, but more people are developing heart disease than ever before. Perhaps still more alarming is the increasing number of young people falling victim to heart disease. In the UK alone, about one in five men, and one in six women die from coronary heart disease, and someone has a heart attack every two minutes. It is the most common cause of premature death in the UK, yet many deaths from heart disease are avoidable. In 2004, 216,000 people in the UK died as a result of heart disease. Perhaps 30,000 more might still be alive if there were no trans fats in our diet.

Are you at risk?

You especially need to know about trans fats if:

- You already have, or are at risk of, coronary heart disease.
- You have had, or are at risk of having, a stroke.
- You are aware that you have high levels of LDL cholesterol.
- You suffer from raised blood pressure (hypertension).
- You have Type 1 or Type 2 diabetes, syndrome X, or any other symptom of insulin resistance.
- You are overweight or obese, especially if you are of the 'apple' rather than 'pear' shape.
- You are trying to get pregnant or are already pregnant.
- You have children and/or are breast-feeding.
- You are not very active in your daily life.

- You are healthy, fit and happy and just want to stay that way!

The danger of trans fats

Trans fats cannot be metabolised by humans so the danger is unique to us. It did not exist prior to Mr Normann's patented invention in 1909. Our cells are confused. Because these chemically produced molecules seem natural, our bodies fail to reject them. Instead, we let them invade our cell membranes where they begin to damage our inherent capacity to protect ourselves.

Human cells cannot tell the difference between natural and manufactured fats. When we consume any kind of fat, trans or other forms, the molecules are absorbed into our cell membranes. If the fat is an industrially produced one, then it fills the space that healthier fats should occupy. Once the trans fat is in position, it cannot be rejected so the integrity of the cell membrane is compromised. The entire behaviour of the cell alters and this tiny link in the chain of human life, this miniature cuckoo, is empowered to disrupt the whole natural pattern of biological exchange between cells.

This is why even small amounts of trans fat intake can have dramatic effects. There are 210 different types of cells in the human body and it is estimated that the total number of cells is something like 100 trillion, yet surprisingly few of them need to be traumatised to cause problems throughout the entire complex system of inter-relating biological exchanges.

Trans fats and heart disease

Heart disease remains the UK's biggest killer and its prevalence increases in areas of deprivation where the consumption of trans fats tends to be higher. The Harvard School of Public Health estimates that up to 100,000 people die every year in the US from cardiovascular disease caused by eating trans fat rather than vegetable oil in its natural state. Although no parallel study has yet been undertaken in the UK, it is reasonable to deduce from the

American study that trans fats here are probably killing up to 30,000 people each year in the UK.

The biggest study to prove the link between trans fats and heart disease is the Nurses' Health Study, which began in Massachusetts in 1976[4] and was followed up in 1989. More than 120,000 female registered nurses have been followed since the study began.

The findings were shocking: just a 2 per cent increase in trans fat calories would bring a 23 per cent increase in that person's risk of developing coronary heart disease. It would take more than a 15 per cent increase in saturated fat calories to get the same effect. We would need to consume nearly seven times the amount of animal fats like butter and lard to endanger ourselves as much as a tiny increase in trans fat would.

Replacing that 2 per cent of our energy intake from trans fats to non-trans- unsaturated fats more than halves the risk of heart disease. This is a much more dramatic risk reduction than we could gain from cutting our saturated fat intake even by 5 per cent.

Trans fat and the cholesterol myth

Cholesterol has had a bad press. There has been so much misinformation around it that many of us have a totally distorted picture of what it is and what it does. Add in the misinformation about trans fat and it is small wonder there is so much confusion.

We need cholesterol. It is a maker and a repairer with an essential role in forming cell membranes, building hormones and vitamin D. It is the body's natural healing substance and 75 per

---

4 The *Nurses' Health Study*, established in 1976 by D. Frank Speizer, and the Nurses' Health Study II, established in 1989 by Dr Walter Willett, are the most definitive long-term epidemiological studies conducted to date on older women's health. The study has followed more than 120,000 female registered nurses since the mid-1970s to assess risk factors for cancer and cardiovascular disease. The studies are among the largest investigations into risk factors for major chronic diseases in women ever conducted. The studies include clinicians, epidemiologists, and statisticians at the Channing Laboratory. Participating organisations from the Massachusetts medical community include the Harvard Medical School, Harvard School of Public Health, Brigham and Women's Hospital, Dana Farber Cancer Institute, Boston Children's Hospital and Beth Israel Deaconess Medical Center.

cent is manufactured within our own liver and cells. The remaining 25 per cent is taken in through food.

When blood vessels are damaged by free radicals or viruses, or because they are structurally weak, it is cholesterol that goes to the damaged site and repairs it with a wax-like substance. Like everything else in the human body's biochemistry, we need to maintain the right levels of cholesterol. It is when there is too much of the wrong kind that we increase our heart disease risk.

The link between raised cholesterol levels and coronary heart disease has been almost completely rubbished by current experts. Dr Malcolm Kendrick, a long-standing skeptic on the cholesterol thesis, argues that the whole hypothesis should be 'consigned to the dustbin of history'.

He points out that it was 40 years ago, back in 1977, that Dr George Mann referred to the supposed link as the 'Greatest scam in the history of medicine' (*New England Journal of Medicine*).

In 1992, a clinical study of 100,000 women found that: 'The pooled estimated risk for total cardiovascular death in women showed no trend across TC (total cholesterol) levels'. In short, for more than 50 per cent of the world's population – women – raised cholesterol is not a risk factor for heart disease.

Moving to men, it is true that under the age of 50 there does seem to be an association between raised cholesterol levels and heart disease. But after the age of 50, when more than 90 per cent of heart attacks happen, the association disappears.

As Dr Kendrick explains: 'Without chasing too many mad arguments around, the simple fact is that everyone in the West does *not* have a raised cholesterol level. Repeated studies have shown that a perfectly normal, or healthy, cholesterol level lies between about four and six, and lowering it cannot protect against heart disease, otherwise we will have introduced a new concept into medical science: normal is unhealthy and must be treated.'

Medicine, and especially research into heart disease, is apt to fall victim to fashion, and experts don't like to acknowledge that they may have got it wrong. The crucial point about cholesterol is to remember that it is the ratio between LDL and HDL that is important in protecting your heart. The two main types of lipoproteins basically work in opposite directions:

Low-density lipoproteins (LDL) carry cholesterol from the liver to the rest of the body. When there is too much LDL cholesterol travelling around the body, apparently it can get deposited on the walls of the coronary arteries. Because of this, LDL cholesterol is often referred to as the 'bad' cholesterol.

High-density lipoproteins (HDL) carry cholesterol back to the liver, which then processes it for elimination from the body. HDL makes it less likely that excess cholesterol in the body will be deposited in the coronary arteries, which is why HDL cholesterol is often referred to as the 'good' cholesterol.

Cholesterol also has a vital role for stress hormones, the corticosteroids, which help us deal with stress, and protect the body against heart disease and cancer. It is important too for our sex hormones like androgen, testosterone, estrogen and progesterone.

Recent research shows that cholesterol acts as an antioxidant. This is the likely explanation for the fact that cholesterol levels go up with age. As an antioxidant, cholesterol protects us against free radical damage that leads to heart disease and cancer.

Cholesterol is needed for proper function of serotonin receptors in the brain. Serotonin is the body's natural 'feel-good' chemical. Low cholesterol levels have been linked to aggressive and violent behaviour, depression and suicidal tendencies.

Breast milk is especially rich in cholesterol, and contains a special enzyme that helps the baby utilise this nutrient. Babies and children need cholesterol-rich foods throughout their growing years to ensure proper development of the brain and nervous system.

Dietary cholesterol plays an important role in maintaining the health of the intestinal wall. This is why low-cholesterol vegetarian diets can lead to leaky gut syndrome and other intestinal disorders.

Cholesterol is not the cause of heart disease but rather a potent antioxidant weapon against free radicals in the blood, and a repair substance that helps heal arterial damage (although the arterial plaques themselves contain very little cholesterol.)

However, like fats, cholesterol may be damaged by exposure to heat and oxygen. This damaged or oxidized cholesterol seems to promote both injury to the arterial cells as well as a build-up of plaque in the arteries. Damaged cholesterol is found in powdered eggs, in powdered milk (added to reduced-fat milks to give them body), and in meats and fats that have been heated to high temperatures in frying and other high-temperature processes, especially partial hydrogenation – trans fats.

What various studies have discovered is that trans fats not only increase the bad LDL but at the same time decrease the good HDL in our bodies, so that there is a pincer effect; a double whammy.

What are your cholesterol levels?

When it comes to testing for cholesterol, there is lots of debate about how meaningful it is. Cholesterol levels are expressed as millimoles per litre of blood, usually shortened to mmol/litre or mmol/l. The United States uses milligrams per decilitre of blood: mg/dl instead. The current guidelines in the UK state that total cholesterol should be kept under 5mmol/l and that, within the amount, the LDL component should be less than 3mmol/l.

We are told that, ideally, all healthy adults, male and female, should seek a level of between 4 and 5 mmol/l but it's not that simple! There is a new blood cholesterol test that measures the level of C-reactive protein, a plasma protein produced by the liver. This may prove to be more useful than existing tests. In a study of more than 700 nurses, findings showed that those who had the highest trans fat consumption also had blood levels of this protein that were 73 per cent higher than those who consumed the lowest levels of trans fat.

Ideal cholesterol levels

The British Heart Foundation recommends:

- a total cholesterol level under 5 mmol/l.
- an LDL level under 3 mmol/l.
- an HDL level above 1 mmol/l.

Do trans fats make you fat?

In terms of weight gain, trans fats may make us more inclined to put on weight than other types of fat. Although trans fat doesn't actually contain more calories than other types of edible fat, it may be that we store it more efficiently and easily.

A highly regarded study carried out in North Carolina by Kylie Kavanagh at Wake Forest University Baptist Medical Center[5] showed that, even with similar calorie intake, trans fat increases weight gain. A six-year experiment revealed that monkeys fed a trans fat diet gained 7.2 per cent in body weight. They also had 30 per cent more abdominal fat, the classic 'apple' shape associated with a predisposition towards cardiovascular disease. The control group, who consumed the same amount of fat but not as trans fat, gained only 1.8 per cent.

Many elements contribute to weight gain and to difficulty in losing weight: a leisurely lifestyle, unhealthy food choices, and unwillingness to take exercise, all play a part. Genetics will tend to influence the likelihood of weight gain, and there are some clinical conditions such as thyroid dysfunction that will impact upon weight. Certain drugs – especially steroids – will encourage weight gain.

In our fast-food era with its associated lack of physical activity, trans fats are an additional problem. Perhaps it is just coincidence that we did not have an obesity epidemic in the west when we did not have trans fat in our foods, but the likelihood of some sort of causal connection is strong.

Do trans fats give you cancer?

The truth is, we still don't really know for sure whether trans fats play any part in the development of cancer. Not enough clinical work has yet been carried out. One study by experts at the Harvard School of Public Health in America does suggest a link between trans fats and prostate cancer in men. Two different

5 Six years of fast-food fats supersizes monkeys *New Scientist Issue* 2556 17 June 2006, page 21

studies reached virtually opposite conclusions on a link with breast cancer, with one saying there was no link and one saying there could be a link.

What is now known comes from research conducted at the University of Maryland and followed up with a later study by Dr Mary Enig, one of the first scientists to sound the alarm about trans fats back in the 1970s. She found that:

> 'trans fatty acids induce adverse alterations in the activities of the important enzyme system that metabolizes chemical carcinogens and drugs (medications), that is, the mixed-function oxidase cytochromes P-448/450.
>
> 'The initial research in this area was done by the Maryland group in collaboration with the US Food and Drug Administration, and was followed by the more extensive evaluation that I did for my PhD dissertation; several groups around the country and the world also reported the same or similar results. Several groups around the world reported a higher intake of partially hydrogenated fats in those individuals who have developed cancer.'

In layman's terms, this means that Dr Enig found a link between trans fat intake and our ability to destroy potential cancer-causing chemicals in our bodies.

A different study by Dr Lenore Kohlmeier[6] studied 700 women, 300 of them with breast cancer, from the United States, the Netherlands, Northern Ireland, Spain, Switzerland, Germany and Finland. The findings reveal an almost 40 per cent increased risk of breast cancer among the women who had higher levels of trans fatty acids stored in their bodies. Samples of tissue taken from the women's buttocks revealed the higher levels of trans fats present. All of the women were post-menopausal, aged between 50 and 74, and researchers controlled the trial statistically for smoking, breast cancer family history, drinking, obesity,

6 Transfat and Breast Cancer, Dr Lenore Kohlmeier, Professor of epidemiology and nutrition at the University of North Carolina 1997

the age at which each woman first gave birth and other habits or conditions that might bias the outcome.

Dr Kohlmeier would like to see further research to confirm the findings: 'This work, because it is the first to show a significant association between breast cancer and trans fatty acids, needs to be confirmed with other studies. Still, we think it is important because so many women are at risk of breast cancer, and there are so few factors, especially dietary factors, known to reduce the risk.'

The Danish Nutrition Council's report from 1995[7] concluded that there was no evidence that dietary levels of trans fatty acids had any carcinogenic effect. Its authors saw no reason to revise that conclusion 10 years later when they called for a ban but advised continued watchfulness regarding any such link.

Trans fats and Type II Diabetes

Most people perceive Type II diabetes only as a less serious form of insulin-dependent Type I diabetes, but in fact, it is an almost entirely different condition. In Type I, which generally emerges in childhood or early adulthood, the ducts in the pancreas that produce the blood glucose controlling hormone, insulin, simply cease to operate. The individual produces absolutely no insulin and blood glucose levels rise rapidly. Thirst and frequent urination are quickly followed by weight loss, exhaustion and sometimes a temporary paralysis if diagnosis is not made promptly. The onset is therefore quite dramatic and failure to recognise the symptoms has the potential to be fatal.

For these people, insulin by injection, through a continuous insulin infusion pump or by inhalation, becomes not just a way of life but life itself. Without insulin every few hours, Type I diabetics will die in a matter of days. There is no alternative, for the moment at least, to putting insulin directly into the blood stream. Taken by mouth, the stomach acids destroy the hormone before it can do its job. The incidence of those with Type I remains fairly static.

7 The influence of trans fatty acids on health, Steen Stender and Jorn Dyerberg, Danish Nutrition Council 1995

But the exponential rise in the incidence of diabetes is in the Type II form. In 2000, there were an estimated 177 million diabetics in the world and by 2025, the number is expected to have increased to 300 million. At least 90 per cent of these individuals will have the Type II condition. More than 80 per cent of the diabetic population will die of cardiovascular disease or stroke.

With Type II diabetes, insulin is still being produced, but it is unable to work properly; the insulin does not lower the blood glucose level appropriately.

It seems that at least some Type II diabetics, far from producing inadequate insulin to meet their needs, may be producing too much. While reduced production, where it occurs, can be stimulated with oral drugs (not insulin) and blood glucose levels brought into the normal zone, over-production and ensuing insulin resistance is a more difficult challenge.

Somehow, the body has lost the capacity to know how to use insulin properly. Although it would be dangerous to make too direct a cause-and-effect connection, there is undoubtedly compelling evidence to link trans fat intake to the human body's inability to maintain proper blood glucose levels.

We know that trans fatty acids disrupt cellular function and stiffen the cell membrane. They affect enzymes and interfere with how we handle both omega-6 and omega-3 essential fatty acids. The amino acids we need to make insulin work properly are disrupted by trans fats. We produce abnormal proteins that cannot handle the insulin properly. The insulin we produce becomes ineffective and Type II diabetes can result. The body produces more and more insulin to try to lower blood glucose but it no longer works.

The Nurses' Health Study (see above) clinicians concluded that increased trans fat intake 'could adversely affect glucose metabolism and insulin resistance.' They found trans fat intake was positively associated with the incidence of Type II diabetes by a factor of up to 39 per cent points.

Giving a high fat meal to the nurses, made up of different kinds of fatty acids, revealed that elaidic acid (a trans fat) gave rise to higher insulin levels in the blood at the same blood sugar level than did the non-trans oleic acid. This finding indicates that elaidic acid produces increased insulin resistance that in turn supports the theory that trans fats promote Type II diabetes.

Although the research picture on the link with Type II diabetes is patchy, the sheer scale and resulting credibility of the Nurses' Health Study gives it a strong standing among professionals. The findings justify the suspicion that a higher intake of trans fat increases the risk of developing Type II diabetes. It does not, so far as we know, have any impact upon those individuals who develop Type I diabetes.

Dr Mary Enig's work in the late 1970s at the University of Baltimore uncovered the link with diabetes. Incidentally, she was not in the pay of any commercial interest. Some groups have expressed the view that the 'diabetes industry' wants to suppress information that might reduce the number of Type II diabetics to whom they can sell everything from glucose monitoring equipment to 'diabetic' chocolate and artificial sweeteners.

The fact remains that trans fats increase blood insulin levels in humans in response to the glucose load, thus increasing the risk factors to health.

Trans fats and allergies

The increased incidence of hay fever, eczema and asthma is considered, by most health professionals, to be connected with our lifestyle. That is, as we become more sedentary, spend less time out of doors, and eat more highly refined and processed food, we are paying the consequences in the increasing number of people experiencing these symptoms.

In 1998, a study of asthma and allergies in childhood (ISSAC) was investigated in 155 centres around the world. They studied the incidence of asthma, allergic cold and asthmatic eczema in children aged 13-14. A positive association was found between the intake of trans fatty acids and these symptoms. Although the information from this investigation does not give guidance on what might be low enough levels of trans fats to avoid these kinds of reactions, it would seem worthwhile to remove trans fats from a child's diet, and see if symptoms improve.

Trans fats and pregnancy

For women seeking to get pregnant, one study showed that a 2 per cent increase in trans fat consumption led to a 73 per cent reduction in ovary infertility (see page 39). One convincing piece of clinical research indicates that a pregnant woman's intake of trans fat is directly manifested in her unborn baby, not least in a reduced birth weight. Previously, it was thought that trans fats did not travel across the uterine wall, but it now seems this information is probably wrong and in fact it does do so.

Women who are breast-feeding should definitely avoid trans fats.

Trans fats and inflammation

There have been two pieces of research that revealed a direct connection between the intake of trans fats and systemic inflammation among women. What this means is that consumption of trans fats will make a woman more likely to experience the pain and discomfort of various kinds of inflammation, especially if she is overweight. Those who already suffer from any kind of inflammation may well discover that cutting out trans fats has a positive effect on an existing condition.

Inflammation is the human body's response to injury and it plays a key role in forming the fatty blockages in blood vessels of the heart. Trans fat damages the cells that line those blood vessels, leading to inflammation.

More health risks

Recent and ongoing research is also investigating the links between trans fats and the following:

1. Liver dysfunction
2. Alzheimer's
3. Some forms of autism and attention-deficit hyperactivity disorder (ADHD)
4. Migraine
5. Hay fever
6. Acid indigestion
7. Vaginal infections
8. Hot flushes
9. Sudden Adult Death Syndrome
10. Nutritional deficiencies – especially a deficiency of omega-3 essential fatty acids

Consumer power

In business everywhere, fear talks. The food industry is starting to spend millions (around £1.5 billion a year at the last estimate) on reformulating their ingredients structure to reduce, and, hopefully, ultimately remove trans fats.

At last, and not before time, the food industry is starting to listen. Extensive pressure created by the lobby organisation Tfx, (www.tfx.org.uk), whose founder, Oliver Tickell, is determined to see all trans fats removed from food ingredients, is starting to see results.

Five grams of trans fat a day increases the risk of heart disease from 4 to 28 per cent. One slice of commercially produced cake could contain four times that amount.

It will take a lot of pressure for the food manufacturers to alter recipes for everything from Horlicks to Haliborange, from muffins to Mars bars. Nestle, Cadbury, GlaxoSmithKline and Marks & Spencer are just some of the big names starting to take an enlightened new approach. Consumer pressure and increasing clinical evidence of the destructive impact is the catalyst for change. Overall, researchers have shown that the damage from trans fats is greater than that caused by food contaminants or pesticide residues.

According to the New England Journal of Medicine study (see page 5), if we eliminated the use of HVOs and used unsaturated oils instead, we could lower the percentage of people suffering from coronary heart disease by up to 22 per cent.

What is the alternative?

Questions are now being asked about the various substitutes that are being used instead of HVOs. Some experts are unconvinced that the alternatives represent any improvement at all. Mono- and di-glycerides are the most widely used of emulsifiers in food production. They crop up in bread, bagels, muffins, cookies, cakes, pies, doughnuts, pasta, potato crisps, ice cream, packaged desserts and most margarines and spreads. There will be some manufacturers who will try to dispute that they are trans fats by describing them as emulsifiers, but they are *trans* and not *cis* in formation.

While the mention on the ingredients list might not sound like trans fat, that is exactly what it is. Mono- and di-glycerides are hydrogenated fats. They are manufactured from glycerin and fatty acids, which are normally obtained from hydrogentaed soya bean oil. We will need to stay very cautious and very alert if we are to avoid substituting one kitchen killer for another one.

There is no such thing as a 'safe level' of trans fat. The only safe level is zero. When we consider that a portion of chips could have 5 grams of trans fat; a doughnut 3 grams, and a small pork pie another 5 grams, we begin to see how much trans fat can be eaten in one day. Across the world, even the most dilatory of countries have accepted that more than 1-2 grams of trans fat is dangerous. The more health-conscious nations, conspicuously the Danes, have agreed that the only acceptable quantity of artificial trans fat is virtually zero. The Danish government has banned the use of hydrogenated vegetable oil anywhere in the food production process.

CHAPTER 4

THE DANGERS OF TRANS FATS FOR CHILDREN

'This will be the first generation where children die before their parents as a consequence of childhood obesity,' warned the House of Commons Health Select Committee in 2004. It is an alarming fact and one that is closely linked to our increased tendency to turn to highly processed convenience foods rather than cooking from scratch. The conflicting demands of work and children have made our lives a struggle in which we do our best to try to balance opposing needs. While we eat out more often than any previous generation, we do not eat better quality food. In fact we eat more fast food than ever before and our children are paying the price.

Weight gain and Type II diabetes used to be the province of middle-aged adults: not so today. These two conditions, often occurring together, are rapidly becoming the hallmark of today's youth. Diabetic specialists are now regularly diagnosing Type II diabetes in young teenagers and sometimes even in primary school age children. In the US, the incidence of Type II among the under 30s has increased by 79 per cent. Why? What has happened that a condition once associated with the over 50s is now striking our children?

The answer is logical if no less alarming for that: our children are living as if they were middle-aged adults and they are paying the price. They are sedentary; they graze constantly on highly processed foods and they are becoming more obese. By 2020, more than half of British children will be overweight.

The message is as stark as it is clear: these are the conse-quences of poor nutrition in childhood. In spite of the admirable efforts of people like Jamie Oliver with his *Jamie's School Dinners* series and a range of initiatives on health promotion, our children continue to pile on the pounds.

We now have two epidemics that go hand-in-hand: Type II diabetes and obesity. The cure will not be found in vaccinations or even in medical advances. Rather, it is entirely in our own hands. The way to change the trend is a healthier lifestyle, one that not only improves general fitness but also provides our children with the nutrients they need and removes our over-reliance on pre-packed and takeaway foods. We have a choice and we need to make that choice with the health of our children in mind.

Good health starts at conception

We have recognised the importance of not smoking and of reduc-ing alcohol intake to virtually zero during pregnancy, yet we carry on eating foods that are damaging to the unborn baby.

Research has shown that trans fats pass between a mother and her unborn baby. This, in turn, inhibits the formation of long-chain polyunsaturated fatty acids (LCPUFAs). Since LCPUFAs are important for both growth and the development of vision and the central nervous system early in life, it is reasonable to conclude that we may be, unwittingly, inflicting damage to an unborn child.

The link to fertility

Fertility may be compromised when correlated with high trans fat intake. In one study, researchers from the Harvard School of Public Health in Boston looked at 18,500 women trying to con-ceive and found 438 cases of problems related to ovulation.

The scientists found that those who took two per cent of their energy intake from trans fats rather than from carbohydrates or polyunsaturated fats had a 70 per cent greater risk of infertility through lack of ovulation. In an average diet, two per cent of energy intake from trans fat could be the result of a daily dough-nut or a couple of sausage rolls.

The link to pre-eclampsia

Another study in 1998 showed that women who developed the life-threatening condition, pre-eclampsia, had a 30 per cent higher level of trans fats in their bloodstream than those who did not.

The link to premature birth

In 1992, a study of premature babies found a negative correlation between birth weight and trans fat levels in plasma four days after birth. Another study in 2001 showed an inverse relationship between the duration of the pregnancy and the level of trans fat in the mother's blood. In other words, high trans fat levels in the mother could mean a premature baby with all the risks attached. More work is being done to try to better define the links, but for anyone seeking to get pregnant, there seems more than adequate evidence already that avoiding trans fats will be good news for the baby.

Breast-feeding mothers should also bear in mind that the trans fats in their bloodstream will continue to be passed on to the baby through breast milk.

Children with Type II diabetes

In terms of the Type II diabetes epidemic (see also page 38), trans fats are playing a dual role. On the one hand, their presence in our diet is directly adding to the number of cases diagnosed because of the links with insulin resistance and obesity. On the other, we know that trans fats increase the risk of cardiovascular disease. Given that people with diabetes are already at an increased risk level of this complication, the addition of trans fat is literally throwing fat onto the fire. Where young people develop both types of diabetes, the risk of heart disease in later life is substantial, so it makes sense to do everything practicable to limit that risk.

Filling up with the wrong foods

Poor levels of nutrition cause other damage too. Oxford University research fellow, Alex Richardson, found between half and two-thirds of children in every age group are getting less than adequate vitamin A in their diet, and 75 per cent of boys and 87 per cent of girls are deficient in vitamin B2. These missing vitamins and minerals have an impact on cell renewal, growth, concentration and energy levels.

What you can do today

Children hate being different. The pressure from peers is intense. It applies in food, schoolwork, sport and leisure as well as in the increasing levels of drug and alcohol abuse. If we are to coax children away from their computer games and onto real, physical games that burn up calories; away from highly processed fast food and towards more natural products, then we need to be clever about it.

Healthy eating for the family:
- Seek a balanced diet for children that will provide them with essential nutrients by giving them fresh food, prepared at home, without the additives that are in pre-packed, processed and takeaway foods.
- A healthy diet includes moderate amounts of chicken and red meat (150g per person, 3 or 4 times a week) as well as oily fish (salmon, mackerel, sardines, herring) a few times a week. Ensure that it is not deep fried in HVO or coated with sauces and dressings that contain it.
- If the household includes vegetarians, make sure they get adequate protein, vitamins and minerals from whole grains (wholemeal flour, brown rice, barley, oats, Shredded Wheat, Weetabix), nuts, cheese, eggs, yoghurt etc. But check ingredient lists to make sure no HVOs have been used.
- Go organic as far as possible.

- Choose meat wisely. Look for grass-fed beef which is rich in omega-3 fatty acids and does not have the overload of omega-6 that corn-fed cattle do. Seek out products without antibiotics or hormones added.
- Cut out in-store bakery products and pre-packed cakes and buns unless you are absolutely certain they contain no trans fats. Bake your own; it's cheaper, more nourishing and the kids enjoy the process.
- Seek out trans fat-free substitutes for crisps, chips, and other favourites. There are plenty of snack alternatives but beware of 'health' or 'energy' bars which can contain partially hydrogenated oil as well as a lot of sugar and additives.
- Be clever with presentation. The child who refuses an unpeeled orange may be happy with a small dish of freshly cut mixed fruit.
- Avoid frying, especially deep frying; it is far better to grill or steam food. Where frying is essential, use groundnut or peanut oil rather than corn or sunflower. The refining process for most of the vegetable oils that we use includes heating to high temperatures, and the balance of nutrients in different oils varies a lot. Best of all are cold-pressed virgin olive oil and walnut oil. Corn, sunflower, soybean and cottonseed oils all contain over 50 per cent omega-6 and, except for soybean oil, only minimal amounts of omega-3. Safflower oil contains almost 80 per cent omega-6. Researchers are just beginning to discover the dangers of excess omega-6 oils in the diet, whether rancid or not. Use of these oils should be strictly limited. They should never be consumed after they have been heated, as in cooking, frying or baking.
- Become aware of appropriate portion sizes for children and teenagers. We generally eat portions that are far larger than we require.
- Be careful when selecting fruit juice drinks. Many of these are made with a lot of sugar and water and very little real juice, so check the ingredients.
- Keep your daily fat intake down to no more than a third of your daily calories. This third needs to be mainly poly- and

monounsaturates. Try to avoid trans fats altogether; not more than a gram or two should be trans fats.

- Avoid unnecessary additives that may cause ADHD, asthma, aggression and poor concentration. The most likely offenders are Tartrazine (E102), Ponceau 4R (E124), Sunset yellow (E110), Carmoisine (E122), Quinoline yellow (E104), Allura red AC (E129), Sodium benzoate (E211), Sodium dioxide (E220), and Sodium metabisulphite (E223).
- If your children won't eat oily fish, introduce omega-3 fish oil capsules into their diet. Other food sources of omega-3 include freshly ground wholegrain cereals, flax and hemp oil seeds, and green leafy vegetables.

Make life easier for you and your family

There is no need to make massive or even very obvious changes to a family's meals to get rid of trans fats and over-processed foods. Substitute a weekly 'treat' of a Kentucky-style bucket of chicken and its 28 grams of trans fats with, for example, roasted chicken legs cooked without hydrogenated fats.

Nor do foods like pizza need to be obliterated. Choose one that has no HVOs or questionable colourings and other artificial additives. Better still, make your own from scratch. In fact, make six and freeze them with just the tomato and cheese base so that other toppings can be added easily before baking in a hot oven for 10 minutes.

Invest in good quality lean, organic meat and poultry. Make chilli con carne, shepherd's pie, lasagne and moussaka at the weekend and freeze in tinfoil trays that are handy for thawing and heating up.

Food need not, and should not, be a battleground for any family. If a child hates cabbage, there is little point trying to force it on him. Look for an alternative. He may like broccoli or he may be content with cabbage that is 'hidden' in fresh minestrone soup or coleslaw. Allowing food to become a divisive issue simply transfers power to the children who are subject to the very peer pressures we are seeking to negate.

Where a main course family dish has been rejected, offer a

basic alternative that is nutritionally sound but do not offer to make an entirely new meal that plays to the fast-food preference. For example, offer cheese or poached egg on toast, cereal, nuts or fruit. If these meet another rejection, try not to vent frustration that may create a full-scale drama. Instead, carry on with the meal and make the alternatives available later on.

Children in the western world, as we have observed, are not in danger of starvation. If a child misses a meal, he will not be in danger of malnutrition. It is worthwhile making breakfast a priority since these calories will contribute to the morning's concentration level at school.

Crucial to success in shifting the nutritional balance at home is the 'buy-in' of the whole family. Convincing children that they will feel healthier, more energetic and will concentrate better provides incentives that will appeal to them. Encourage them to participate in the changes and to find alternatives to, for example, biscuits and crisps that contain trans fats. Get them reading the long ingredients lists that reveal the vast amounts of junk we are all eating and ask them to find products that won't poison them.

Preparing food at home can sound like hard work, but there are ways of minimising the effort:

- Use the freezer. Home-frozen food preserves most of the nutritional value.
- Use raw food. Fruit and vegetables don't necessarily require cooking.
- Don't bother peeling vegetables. A thorough wash is all that's needed, especially when using organic produce that will not have chemical additives. Much of the best vitamin content of potatoes and carrots, for example, is just under the skin and is lost by peeling.
- Use a slow cooker. This form of cooking protects the nutrients and makes it practical to come home to a meal that is fully cooked without requiring any attention during the day.
- Use a juicer. For children who are not good at eating fresh fruit and vegetables, a juicer is a quick and easy way of

producing an alternative that, while it loses some of the fibre content, preserves the vitamin and mineral content.

- Use pulses in soups and pasta sauces. Some pulses need overnight soaking so pre-planning is necessary, but others, such as lentils, are quick and easy to cook. The Indian staple, dahl, is easy to make.
- Provide snack foods that are a healthy alternative to crisps and confectionery. Dried apricots, nuts, flax and hemp seeds, pumpkin seeds, fresh fruit, vegetable sticks and wholegrain crackers, for example.

CHAPTER 5

GETTING TRANS FATS OUT OF YOUR LIFE

You can eliminate trans fats from your food. It is well within your own power to remove this potential killer from your life. Buying food without buying trans fats will benefit everyone. We can each play a part in moving towards a trans fat-free world in which fewer people are dying from avoidable causes. Unlike some threats we may face, this is one you can control and remove.

Here is some guidance to help you avoid consuming partially hydrogenated oils. What is here will not strip out every source of trans fats, but as your awareness and experience increase, you will find that you develop a powerful intuition about the kinds of foods most likely to contain trans fats. You will be better equipped to avoid them and opt for healthier choices.

A word of warning: getting rid of trans fats is not a license to replace them with saturated fats! While butter is better than trans fat-laden margarine, for example, it would be no kindness to your health to overload your system with saturated fats, however natural they are.

There is no single group of prepared foods that we can avoid completely and therefore cut out every source of trans fat. Because trans fats are used in so many food products, avoiding them requires a more consistent and thorough approach but it definitely pays to be suspicious, particularly when it comes to in-store baked or takeaway food without any ingredients information.

Most of the trans fats in a typical Western diet comes from

commercially baked and fried foods that are made with vegetable shortening, some margarine (especially hard margarines), or oils containing partially hydrogenated oils and fats. French fries, doughnuts, pastries, muffins, croissants, cookies, crackers, crisps and other snack foods are high in trans fatty acids. In fact, many fried or baked goods in the UK will contain some trans fats, perhaps with up to 50 per cent of the total fat content. A great deal of confectionery also includes hydrogenated vegetable oil.

As manufacturers gradually shift away to alternatives, we cannot necessarily be very reassured since many are using hydrogenated rapeseed, coconut and palm oil. There is also an increased usage of mono-glycerides and di-glycerides (MGs and DGs). These are usually by-products from the processing – including partial hydrogenation – of various oils and fats.

Though they do have some caloric value, MG and DG are not classed as fats so even if there are *trans* bonds in there, they won't be identified as such on the ingredients panel.

As people become more aware of hydrogenated oils, food manufacturers are likely to use MGs and DGs containing trans fats more and more, to get that famous 'mouth feel.' They won't need to say anything about that in the ingredients or on the nutrition panel. We will need to remain watchful.

Mono-glycerides and di-glycerides are actually normal constituents in the digestion of food fats, but the MGs and DGs listed on the labels of our foods are constructed from fats and oils and used as surfactants to make it easier for companies to make their products.

Research in November 2007 revealed that hydrogenated vegetable oil was still listed as an ingredient in the following food items:

- Knorr stock cubes
- Mr Kipling Chocolate Chip Cake bars
- Krispy Kreme doughnuts
- Snickers bar
- Twix bar
- Jacob's Tuc crackers

- Bird's Eye potato waffles
- Nestle Quality Street
- Mars Maltesers
- Mars Revels
- Mars Celebrations
- Mars M+Ms
- Maynard's wine gums
- Halo Fairtrade Honey, Raisin and Chocolate cereal bars
- Elmlea artifical cream
- Bachelor's Cuppa Soup
- Sainsbury's frozen cod in butter sauce
- Horlicks drinks
- Haliborange omega-3 fish oils for children
- Tulip Cheese and Bacon Grills
- Lees Mini-snowballs and Snowcakes
- Crosse & Blackwell Bonne Cuisine Bechamel Sauce mix
- Old El Paso Original Enchiladas
- Maltesers Instant hot chocolate drink
- Cadbury Instant hot chocolate drink
- Betty Crocker Premium Icing
- Cadbury 'Snowie Snowman' cake mix
- Jane Asher Rich Fruit Christmas Cake mix
- Angel Delight dessert

The list is by no means inclusive and is provided just to give a flavour of some of the familiar foods that contain trans fats. There are many more. While the eight supermarket chains – Asda, Boots, Co-op, Iceland, Waitrose, Marks & Spencer, Sainsbury's and Tesco – had all committed to removing HVOs completely from their own-brand ranges by the end of 2007, there is scant evidence of food manufacturers in the UK seeking ways to eliminate their use across all the familiar brand names.

Read the labels

Study the ingredients lists on food labels and you will find that HVO finds its way into thousands of everyday foods, including many with a 'healthy' image, such as cereal bars, low-fat biscuits and vegetarian burgers. Even toddler and infant foods can contain it.

If the term 'hydrogenated' appears anywhere in the ingredients list, put the product back on the shelf and seek an alternative. Get the children involved in this mission and send them around the supermarket aisles to find foods that do not list hydrogenated vegetable oil as an ingredient. Check store cupboard foods at home and dispense with those that contain trans fats. They will be there in everything from soups to sweets and biscuits to beef stew.

Here are a few sample ingredients lists from products currently on sale in the UK:

WAFER WITH NOUGAT CREAM AND MILK CHOCOLATE
Ingredients: sugar, wheat flour, **hydrogenated vegetable fat**, cocoa butter, hazelnuts 9.8%, cocoa mass, skimmed milk powder, whey powder, lactose, butterfat, whey product, low-fat cocoa powder, milk powder, emulsifier (lecithins), flavouring, invert sugar syrup, salt, raising agent (sodium hydrogen carbonate).

CHOKO PLESKNER: BISCUITS WITH COCOA BASE
Ingredients: Wheat flour, sugar, **margarine (partially hydrogenated vegetable fat)**, water, salt, milk protein, lactose, emulsifiers (E471, E322), acidity regulator: citric acid. Flavouring: **partially hydrogenated vegetable fat**, whole eggs, low-fat cocoa (3%), full-cream milk powder, raising agents (E450, E500), emulsifier (E322).

CHOCOLATE SWISS ROLL WITH VANILLA-FLAVOURED CREAM
Ingredients: vanilla-flavoured cream 33.3% **(partially hydrogenated vegetable oil)** and vegetable oil, glucose syrup, lactose, emulsifier: E471; vanilla flavouring, wheat flour, sugar, pasteurised eggs, glucose syrup, low-fat cocoa powder 2%, lactose, stabilisers: E420, E422; emulsifiers: E471, E475; milk powder, white Vekao icing (contains emulsifier: E322), raising agents: E450, E500; salt, vanilla flavouring, cocoa flavouring, acid: E260, citric acid. This product may contain traces of nuts.

*

Most of the trans fats we consume come from unlabelled produce, whether that is in a café or restaurant or in a takeaway
lunch pack, so the supermarket shop actually gives us more control. Our purchasing power as consumers is worth exploiting. If
supermarkets are convinced that rejecting supplies with trans
fat in their ingredients will reap benefits, then they will do it. If
the suppliers are in turn pressurised by their big customers, they,
too, will respond by finding alternatives.

Strides in food technology now mean that there are safe alternatives. Even JM Smucker, the owner of the Crisco brand, has
managed to reformulate its iconic product without HVOs and
with only traces of trans fats.

What is your family eating?

One doughnut a day is enough to increase the risk of developing
coronary heart disease by 23 per cent. If a typical family is consuming biscuits, commercially baked cake, dried soup and
perhaps instant gravy granules a few times a week, then each
member could be eating 10 grams of trans fat in a single day. Add
a deep-fried chicken meal or a burger and chips and the amount
could be trebled. Why not look through your cupboards and
fridge and work out what your family is really eating. It is clear
that trans fats are not the preserve of couch-potato junk food
addicts. While experts are still debating what constitutes a 'safe'
level of trans fat intake, and many opt for zero, the generally
conceded maximum is two grams a day.

How to eat zero trans fats

There are plenty of foods that don't contain any trans fats so we
can start with these:

- All fresh fruit and vegetables
- Fresh meat, fish and chicken

- Tinned fish, fruit and vegetables
- Milk, butter and yoghurt
- Honey
- Cheese, providing that it has not been processed with hydrogenated oils
- Fresh eggs
- Uncooked grains and pasta
- Fruit juices and fruit drinks
- Dried fruit and nut mixes

There is a group of foods that generally do not contain trans fats but sometimes do. Read the labels on:

- Commercially baked pre-packaged bread
- Chutneys, pickles, olives
- Fresh soup packaged in cartons/plastic bottles
- Vegetables prepared in an oil dressing
- Hot chocolate or malted bedtime drinks
- Jams and marmalades
- Roasted nuts

And the most likely supermarket offenders of all are:

- In-store bakery produce from supermarkets which have not yet removed hydrogenated vegetable oil products – bread, pizza bases, croissants, Danish pastries, fondants, cheesecakes, birthday cakes
- Salad bars (the HVOs tend to be in the dressing)
- Salad dressings
- Most deep-fried foods
- Pastry goods such as pies and quiches (savoury and sweet)
- Chocolate and peanut butter spreads
- Pudding mixes
- Pre-packaged cakes with a long shelf-life
- Doughnuts
- Biscuits and cookies (both in-story bakery and pre-packaged)
- Lots of confectionery designed specifically to appeal to children

- Many children's cereals, even where marketed as 'nutritious' or 'wholesome'
- Many frozen foods, especially potato waffles and chips but also many prepared meals
- Frozen desserts and tarts
- Some ice cream, especially economy varieties
- Ready-made chilled meals
- Dried soup and stuffing mixes
- Dehydrated stock powders, granules and cubes
- Savoury crackers and snack products
- Potato crisps and associated snack products
- Bakery mixes
- Bakery decorating and icing products
- Cake fillings
- Sandwich fillings
- Sauce mixes

The simplest and most effective rule of thumb when buying supermarket food is to buy organic and always cook from scratch. If we reject pre-packed, processed foods, we will not be consuming trans fats. Of course, life is not quite so straightforward and pressures of time and family can mean we sometimes resort to fast foods in some shape or form.

But fast foods do not have to be processed foods. Fruit and cheese with fresh wheaten bread is virtually instant and completely without artificial additives, especially if we purchase organically grown products that will be free from chemical pesticides and fertilisers. If the family want burgers, avoid the multipacks of economy frozen ones with 'not less than 37% meat' and either buy ready-made, organically produced burgers or make them at home.

We need to be open to alternatives and to think about the week ahead before going shopping. That way, with a little forward planning, it is easy to buy raw ingredients that can be used to make a number of different dishes.

Why we should buy organic produce

The good news is that it is becoming easier every day to buy high-quality food that does not contain potentially dangerous additives.

The grain-based diet that most commercially bred livestock is fed on does nothing to improve either its health-giving potential for us nor the quality of life for the animal. Our farmed animals evolved to eat grass but even in something as basic as this, humans have decided that we know better. And since when did a wire cage for three or four birds masquerade as the perfect environment for the production of good quality, fresh eggs?

We are beset by relentless advertising that tells us our environment isn't clean enough and that we should be spraying anti-bacterial products on every surface, and peeling every carrot, apple or potato to ensure that it can't infect us. We are sold concoctions to discourage viruses and attack bacteria, we wear masks to fight off pollution and we panic under health scares, including SARS, bird flu and MRSA. Of course, there are real issues here, but we have distorted them to such an extent that we are creating a new phobia about germs.

Germs have always been with us and in fact our ecology needs them. Without the bacteria in our gut we would be unable to digest our food. Without the various, mainly harmless, bacteria and viruses that fill every breath we take in, we would be unable to create our own immune system. The main fight against the germs we do not want starts and finishes with a very simple protocol: wash your hands thoroughly. That act alone will eliminate most of the potential threat.

So let us shed our fear of leafy vegetables and chickens that look as if they might once have run around a farmyard. Let us get rid of the unnecessary packaging, cling film and polystyrene containers that do us, and our environment, harm. Let's start buying the actual food we want to eat from the producers who sell it as it is. Let's stop looking for cucumbers that are always the same size and thickness, for bananas that are uniform, and apples that look identical.

By and large, we are best served by finding good producers

close to where we live. Fresh food deteriorates rapidly, no matter how carefully it is packaged, and the shorter the gap between harvesting and serving, the better the end product.

The tremendous growth of The Farmers Market network across the country means that there is a weekly outlet close to many of us. Check www.farmersmarkets.net and www.scottish-farmersmarkets.co.uk There are too many local websites to list here. They run from Exeter to Glasgow, from London to Newcastle and cover every district of the UK and Ireland. A quick web search will allow you to identify those nearby. There are also a range of organic supplier directories available. For example, the Organic Directory produced by the Soil Association is available online at: www.whyorganic.org. Each UK region of the Soil Association produces a directory of its own but all are available through the portal www.localfoodworks.org

When shopping online, you will find local outlets who will deliver in your immediate area, but we list here some of the retailers who deliver throughout the country. When it comes to fruit and vegetables, it is especially important to seek out local suppliers. Fresh products are highly perishable and lose much of their valuable mineral and vitamin content very rapidly. The fresher the produce, the better it will be. It is best to use fresh produce like this within a day or two, rather than to keep it for a week.

Organically produced food costs more. The farming methods are more expensive for a range of reasons: it is more labour-intensive, crops are grown less often in the same piece of ground and animals are held at lower stocking densities for their own well-being. The careful controls placed on organic production (including the licensing system) add to the costs of production. Organic farming essentials like seed and animal feed cost more than their non-organic versions. However, the more people demand organic produce, the lower the unit cost becomes. Besides, organic production is not 'costing the earth' in terms of destroying our environment or our health with polluted water and chemical spills.

Organic suppliers

Here is a list of established businesses that, between them, supply organic meat, fish, dairy produce and vegetables. Some will have free delivery. There will be others in your local area so do shop around.

Daylesford Organic
www.daylesfordorganic.com

Graig Farm Organics (also bakery, grocery, dairy and fish)
www.graigfarm.co.uk

Helen Browning Organics
www.helenbrowningorganics.co.uk

Higher Hackness Farm
www.higherhackness.co.uk

Sheepdrove Organic Farm
www.sheepdrove.com

Well Hung Meat
www.wellhungmeat.com

FISH
Inverawe smokehouses
www.smokedsalmon.co.uk

The Organic Smokehouse
www.organicsmokeshouse.com

Deverill Trout Farm
www.purelyorganic.co.uk

Loch Fyne
www.lochfyne.com

Planning the week ahead

While every family will have its preferences when it comes to
meals, we've created a fairly typical sample family here to offer
suggestions on how it's possible to buy healthy, nutritious food
without either spending a fortune or eating a very limited selection of foods.

Fiona and Paul have two children, Hannah is 6 and Patrick is
10. Like many children, they have their own ideas about what
they like but are not unadventurous and they enjoy cooking.
Here's what Fiona buys each week. All the ingredients and
products are organic and free-range. Some items do not need to
be bought each week, for example, olive oil and flour. Average
total cost of the weekly shop for a family of four: approximately
£75

Fresh fruit and vegetables:
Fiona buys a vegetable box each week from a local organic food
supplier which includes seasonal vegetables, fruit and usually
either a cauliflower or a cabbage. Delivered to her door, it costs
£15. There are such suppliers available in many parts of the UK.
This week she supplements it with additional organic potatoes
from the supermarket, a large bunch of bananas and a selection
of seasonal fruit including six apples and two lemons.

Meat and fish:
- A whole free-range corn-fed chicken for Sunday evening
- A tray of free-range chicken thighs and drumsticks
- 1 kg lean steak mince
- 1 kg steak pieces
- 3 cans tuna fish in brine
- 2 fresh trout
- 1 salmon joint

Bakery
- 2 large loaves of sunflower and pumpkin seed bread
- Pack of 10 wholemeal rolls

Dairy
- 500g cheddar cheese
- 100g feta cheese
- 3 ltrs semi-skimmed milk
- 2 ltrs whole milk
- 10 yoghurts in various fruit flavours
- 500g butter
- 12 free range eggs

Store cupboard
- ½ litre olive oil
- 1 litre sunflower oil
- Lasagne sheets
- Couscous
- Small tub of olives
- 4 tins chopped tomatoes
- Cinnamon, nutmeg and vanilla
- 1kg oatmeal
- 1 kg plain flour
- 1 kg Muscavado sugar
- Tomato purée
- Stock cubes
- 1 bottle wine

Here are some of the week's dishes:

Breakfasts
Paul and Patrick both enjoy porridge made with a mix of milk and water, sweetened with honey and with some cold milk on top. Fiona and Hanna prefer wholemeal toast with banana.

Lunches
Both of the children take a packed lunch to school. They have wholemeal rolls with a variety of fillings: tuna, cheese, chicken, salad and egg mayonnaise, for example. She gives each child a piece of fruit and a yoghurt each day. They get water from the cooler at school. For her own lunch, Fiona will have a couscous salad, or a roll or sandwich. She will probably make some

vegetable soup this week. Paul's office has a wholefood sandwich trolley that visits every day.

Supper

Patrick and Paul roasted the chicken on Sunday. They had mashed potatoes and fresh young carrots from the vegetable box. Fiona prepared a lasagne on Saturday which she will serve on Monday. Other main meals during the week will include home-made organic burgers, a slow-cooked casserole of beef, baked salmon, baked potatoes with tuna and a cheese soufflé with salad.

Family favourite recipes

There are lots of ways to prepare the food that the family has purchased but here are some ideas.

All recipes serve 4 unless otherwise stated. All the ingredients are organic.

Whole roast chicken with garlic

This method of roasting a chicken creates a lovely piquancy from the garlic bulb. The honeyed carrots are popular with children.

Ingredients
1 free-range corn-fed chicken
2 tbsp olive oil
1 bulb of garlic, peeled roughly
1.5kg potatoes, peeled
500g carrots, washed
1 tbsp honey
A little milk and butter
Black pepper and salt, to season

Method
1. Heat the oven to 180°C.
2. Rub the outside of the chicken with the olive oil, and season with freshly ground pepper and salt. Place the garlic bulb in the cavity.

3. Roast, basting occasionally, for 1-2 hours, according to the weight of your chicken. When browned and cooked through, set aside to rest, covered to retain the heat.

4. Steam the carrots for a few minutes until tender, then toss them in a little honey and place in the oven for 10 minutes.

5. Meanwhile, boil the potatoes for 10-15 minutes, then drain. Add a little milk and butter to the pan, and mash well with salt and pepper.

6. Serve the chicken with the baked carrots and mashed potatoes.

Beef lasagne

Lasagne is a perennial favourite that can be prepared in advance and freezes well. The slight twist provided by adding spinach or broccoli to half of the sauce introduces some green vegetables and a nice touch of colour, but can be left out if preferred. The wine adds richness to the sauce, but, again, is not essential. You can double the amount of stock that you use instead.

Ingredients
3 cloves of garlic, peeled and crushed
1 medium onion, peeled and chopped
1 large carrot, peeled and chopped
1 tsp fresh or ½ tsp dried oregano
300g organic minced beef
1 can chopped tomatoes
1 tbsp tomato purée
200ml red wine
1 organic chicken stock cube, dissolved in 100ml boiling water
340g organic lasagne sheets
Olive oil
Salt and pepper

For the béchamel sauce
50g butter
50g plain flour
500 ml milk
4-5 whole black peppercorns
120 ml cream

½ tsp ground cinnamon
½ tsp ground nutmeg
A couple of bay leaves
150g cheddar cheese, grated
150g spinach or broccoli (if using broccoli, finely chop the top florets)

Method

1. Use olive oil to grease a large ovenproof dish.

2. Heat 2 tbsps of olive oil in a heavy-based frying pan, then add the garlic and onion. Cook until light golden.

3. Add the carrot, oregano and minced beef. Brown the beef well, breaking up any lumps, and turning the ingredients to blend. After about five minutes, add the tomatoes, tomato purée, wine and stock cube, then season with freshly ground salt and pepper.

4. Simmer gently, half-covered, stirring occasionally, for around 30 minutes. The mixture will reduce. Meanwhile, heat the oven to 180°C.

5. To make the Bechamel sauce, melt the butter in a saucepan over a low heat. Add the flour, stirring constantly with a wire whisk or a fork.

6. Gradually add the milk to the roux, stirring all the time, until the two are blended into a sauce. Add the peppercorns and bay leaves.

7. Simmer the sauce for two minutes to cook the flour, then divide it into two pans. To one, add the cream, cinnamon and nutmeg and half of the grated cheese. Cook until the cheese has melted. Season with salt and pepper. To the other, add the broccoli or spinach and turn both pans off. Remove the bay leaves.

8. Now cook the pasta sheets in a large pan of boiling water with some salt and olive oil added (to stop it from sticking) according to the instructions on the packet – usually about 6 minutes. Fresh sheets and some dried varieties don't require pre-cooking and can be placed straight into the baking dish.

9. To assemble the lasagne, spoon half of the spinach/broccoli sauce into the greased ovenproof dish and spread it out evenly. Place a layer of lasagne pasta on top. Spread half the minced

beef mixture evenly over the pasta and cover with another pasta layer.

10. Spread the remaining spinach/broccoli mixture over next, and cover with another layer of pasta. Spread the last of the beef mixture over evenly.

11. Add the last layer of pasta and cover it with the cheese sauce mixture. Spread it out evenly and sprinkle the remaining grated cheese on top.

12. Place in the middle of the preheated oven and cook for around 30 minutes until the top has turned golden brown.

Steak and stout casserole

This is a lovely warming winter meal that can be started in the slow cooker early in the day then left to cook gently without any attention for 8 hours or more. You don't have to use Guinness; any stout will do. The addition of some crème fraiche when serving is nice.

If you don't have a slow cooker, you can cook this dish in an ovenproof casserole dish. The casserole is delicious served with baked or mashed potatoes.

Ingredients
1kg steak pieces
A little flour and mustard powder
One large onion, peeled and roughly chopped
Olive oil, for frying
2 bay leaves
½ teaspoon dried herbs of your choice
1 small can or bottle of Guinness or stout
20 shallots, peeled
3 large carrots, peeled and cut into large chunks
3 parsnips, peeled and cut into large chunks
2 organic beef stock cubes dissolved in 200 ml of boiling water

Method
1. Toss the steak pieces in a bowl containing the flour, mustard, salt and pepper, until well-coated.
2. Fry the onion in the olive oil for two minutes until softened,

then add the steak, a few pieces at a time, until it is browned all over.

3. Transfer the steak and onions to the slow cooker or casserole dish. Toss the shallots, carrots and parsnips in the pan oil and add these to the meat. Season with salt and pepper, and add the bay leaves and herbs of your choice.

4. Add the stock and Guinness or stout and set the slow cooker on high for a couple of hours before turning to low for around 4-5 hours. Alternatively, cook in a preheated oven at 200°C for 1-2 hours.

Home-made beef burgers

Making burgers at home is quick, easy and far more wholesome than most of what you can buy. You can also use minced pork or lamb or any combination of meats. You can add toppings of cheese, tomato and salad.

Ingredients
500g lean organic beef mince
1 onion, peeled and finely chopped
A bunch of parsley, chopped
1 large egg, beaten
50g breadcrumbs
Olive oil, for frying
4 burger buns to serve
Black pepper and salt, to season
Chopped lettuce, onion and tomato to serve

Method
1. Combine the mince with the chopped onion, parsley, breadcrumbs and season well.

2. Add the beaten egg and shape into four burgers. Grill or shallow fry in olive oil for about six minutes on each side. Serve on warmed burger rolls, topped with chopped salad.

Baked potatoes with tuna mayonnaise

Baking potatoes is fairly slow, so you may like to do a batch that will last over a couple of days, re-heating as required. Simply reheat when needed for about 15 minutes at 190°C. You can make alternative fillings out of weekend leftovers such as chicken, or make a vegetarian option with grated cheese mixed with mayonnaise and spring onions.

Ingredients
4 large baking potatoes
2-3 cans tuna in brine, drained
2 spring onions, finely chopped
4 tbsp mayonnaise (see recipe below)
Black pepper and salt, to season

Method
1. Wash and dry the potatoes, then make small holes in them with a fork. Rub olive oil and salt into each one and place in a hot oven at 200°C for 60-75 minutes, turning half way through.
2. Flake the tuna in a bowl, add the chopped onions and seasoning and combine with the mayonnaise. Serve spooned into the baked potatoes.

Mayonnaise
Commercially prepared mayonnaise and salad dressings often use hydrogenated vegetable oil so the best way to avoid this is to make your own. Homemade mayonnaise is a little time consuming but it is not difficult to make and will keep in the fridge for about a week. You can also add variants: a tablespoon of tomato purée, smoked paprika, chopped capers, or gherkins, for example.

Ingredients
250 ml high-quality, cold-refined vegetable or nut-based oil such as groundnut, sunflower, peanut or olive
2 egg yolks, at room temperature
Juice of one lemon or a little white wine or cider vinegar
Black pepper and salt, to season

Method
1. Whisk the egg yolks with a small wire whisk or a fork. Now

begin adding the oil, just a drop at a time. Once you have combined the first couple of tablespoons, you will have an egg emulsion that gradually thickens as you add more oil.

2. Once it has become thickened, add a dessertspoonful of lemon juice or vinegar to thin the emulsion. Now continue to add more oil. The mayonnaise will gradually thicken up again and you can then add more lemon juice or vinegar to get the consistency you want.

3. Add freshly ground salt and black pepper to taste.

Easy Victoria Sponge

When it comes to home baking, we've rather got out of the habit! I'd like to suggest it's time we bypassed the ready-made counters and baked for ourselves. It doesn't demand a huge amount of time or effort, it's incredibly satisfying, will save you money and when it comes to taste, there's just no comparison.

Ingredients
100g soft trans fat-free margarine
2 free range eggs
100g caster sugar
100g self-raising flour
2 drops pure vanilla essence
2 tbsp raspberry jam
2 tbsp fresh whipped cream (optional)
Icing sugar, to dust

Method
1. Preheat the oven to 180°C. Line two round 7-inch cake tins with greaseproof paper. Brush the paper with sunflower oil.

2. Mix together the margarine and caster sugar. Add the eggs and flour and beat with an electric hand mixer or wooden spoon until smooth.

3. Divide the mixture evenly between the two tins, and bake for 25-30 minutes until golden and risen.

4. Turn out onto a wire rack to cool. When cool, spread one layer with raspberry jam and the other with cream, if using. Sandwich the two together and dust with sieved icing sugar, to serve.

No-fat lemon sponge

A light, tangy cake that tastes indulgent, although it contains hardly any fat.

Ingredients

3 free-range eggs
100g honey
100g self-raising flour
Juice and grated rind of one lemon
2 tbsp lemon curd

Method

1. Heat the oven to 200°C. Line two round 7-inch cake tins with greaseproof paper. Brush the paper with sunflower oil.
2. Separate the eggs and put the whites to one side. Beat the yolks with the honey until thick and creamy. Beat in the flour, lemon juice and rind.
3. In a separate bowl, whisk the egg whites until stiff. Using a metal spoon, fold these into the flour mixture.
4. Divide the mixture between the two tins and bake for 10-15 minutes, until risen.
5. Turn onto a wire rack to cool. When cool, sandwich together using the lemon curd.

Flapjack bars

(makes 12 bars)
You can use any combination of dried fruit and seeds to vary this recipe each time you make it. Store in an airtight container for up to one week. These are useful to drop into a child's school lunch box or fill a gap in the late afternoon.

Ingredients

4 tbsp 100% sunflower oil
6 tbsp honey
25g light Muscovado sugar
150g organic oats
50g sunflower seeds
25g sesame seeds

25g desiccated coconut
50g dried apricot pieces, chopped
50g sultanas

Method
1. Heat the oven to 180°C. Grease an 11x7-inch baking tray with butter or sunflower oil.
2. Combine the oil and honey in a saucepan and heat gently until the honey is melted. Remove from the heat and add all the remaining ingredients. Mix well to combine.
3. Press the mixture into the greased tray and smooth the top. Bake for 20-25 minutes until pale golden.
4. Using a knife, mark into 12 bars while still hot, then leave the tray to cool slightly. Cut into slices and transfer to a wire rack to cool.

Blackberry and apple crumble
You can vary the filling for this crumble, changing the fruit to suit the seasons. Commercially produced crumble topping is one of the regular sources of hydrogenated vegetable oil and trans fat. Making your own is quick and easy as well as cheaper, tastier and more nutritious.

Ingredients
500g cooking apples, peeled, cored and thickly sliced
350g blackberries
50g golden caster sugar
90g butter, cut into cubes
150g plain flour
50g rolled oats
4 tbsp Demerara sugar

Method
1. Heat the oven to 200°C. Lightly grease a shallow pie dish with butter.
2. Layer the apples and blackberries into the dish, sprinkling each layer with the caster sugar.
3. Make the crumble topping by rubbing the cubed butter into

the flour until the mixture resembles coarse breadcrumbs. Stir in the oats and Demerara sugar.

4. Sprinkle the topping over the fruit and bake for 35-40 minutes until the top is crisp and golden.

CHAPTER 6

ACTION AROUND THE WORLD

Denmark is the trail-blazer and the only country in the world to put the shelf-life of its people above the shelf-life of the products we purchase. Denmark banned the use of trans fats throughout the food industry in March 2003. By January 2004, Denmark was the only country in the world where you could be confident that you were unlikely to consume more than a gram of industrially produced trans fat in a day. While the abolition caused some short-term problems for manufacturers seeking substitutes, the Danish food industry did not grind to a halt as a result of the ban. Tens of thousands more Danes are alive today than would be had the ban not been instigated. Don't we all share in that right?

The two main consumer-led websites on the subject of trans fats are:
www.bantransfats.com in the States
and
www.tfx.org.uk in the UK

Denmark leading the way

We have already said that the only safe level of trans fat consumption is none. In the US, under 0.5g per serving can be described as 'zero' and some theorists suggest that under a gram a day won't harm us, but there is no universal agreement about 'safe' levels of trans fats. The Danes have banned trans fats not only in packaged produce but also in the *entire catering and food preparation industry.* Following advice from the Danish Nutrition Council, the Government simply took the view that the health of its people was more important than the health of the food industry and that was that. Even the food industry wasn't horrified and admits that the ban hadn't caused any major problems for them. They have found alternatives or learned to live with some products having a shorter shelf life.

In the UK, we don't take the same view. We have not decided to ban trans fats, regardless of the health risks and the incontrovertible evidence that trans fats can kill. Instead, we call for voluntary regulation and try to persuade the big supermarket chains that it would be a good idea to show a commitment to cutting back on the trans fat content in foods. Some supermarkets seek active public relations gains by saying they're doing everything they can to cut back on the trans fats in their own-brand products. That's all very good and helpful, but why don't they just stop using them now?

What is happening in the UK?

At home, we have been slow to recognise the danger that lurks in HVOs. The risk really intensified in the 1970s when saturated fats were 'out' and a vegetable-based substitute seemed like a good alternative.

Yet our own Food Standards Agency (FSA), which is responsible for food labelling and safety, seems reluctant, more than 25 years later, to really tackle the problem or face down the industry. Bakery products, takeaways and confectionery remain uncontrolled in terms of the trans fats they use in production.

Its website (www.food.gov.uk) says: 'The trans fats found in food containing hydrogenated vegetable oil are harmful and have no known nutritional benefits'. And it advises consumers, 'Cut down on food that is high in saturated fat or trans fats'.

But the FSA does not make manufacturers label the trans fat content of their products. Asked about how consumers are meant to follow their advice to cut back on food high in trans fats, the FSA could only say that trans fats were mostly found in foods such as cakes and biscuits which people shouldn't eat too much of anyway, and that consumers are free to avoid foods containing HVO.

Alex Richardson is senior research fellow at Oxford University's department of physiology, and director of the campaigning charity Food and Behaviour Research. She believes that Britain should follow Denmark, which has had legislation since 2003 limiting the amount of trans fats in food. 'There's nothing to say in trans fats' defence,' she says. 'They appear to be more dangerous than saturated fats, they have no nutritional value, they are an artificial, toxic fat that we don't need. I don't see just why we can't have them out of the food supply. We have a major public-health problem here with diabetes and heart disease, and losing one contributory fat is a step towards the solution'.

At the end of July 2006, the British Medical Journal published a review of a vast amount of disparate research. The most important single fact that has held up is that a 2 per cent rise in our energy intake from trans fatty acids (about 5g of trans fat a day) 'was associated with a 23 per cent increase in the incidence of coronary heart disease' (see also page 26).

In its editorial, the BMJ called on the government to legislate to reduce trans fats to less than 2 per cent of food content (as in Denmark) and to force manufacturers to quantify trans fats on labels (as has been done in the US since the beginning of 2006). The review also highlighted the fact that at least two studies have shown hydrogenation destroys the healthy omega-3 oils, and that eating trans fats may block their uptake.

McDonalds has already been fined by the courts in America for failing to deliver on its promise to remove trans fats in 2003, and many others will shelter behind these voluntary agreements. Only legal statute is likely to really change the situation. McDonald's is to switch to low trans fat frying oils made from high-oleic acid varieties of UK-grown rapeseed. The company prides itself on using local ingredients but has had some difficulties getting sufficient quantities of rapeseed oil lined up. It expected to have rolled out the new oil, which contains 2 per cent or less trans fat, into all its 1,200 outlets by the end of 2007. McDonald's is the first fast food chain in the UK to commit to this kind of move.

However, rapeseed and canola, the most commonly used vegetable oils in the EU, are not without their critics. Rapeseed can contain quite high levels of trans fats. Researchers at the University of Florida at Gainesville found that liquid canola/rapeseed oils sold in the USA contained as much as 4.6 per cent trans fat. The only certain way to find out the trans fat content of your brand of vegetable oil is to write to the manufacturer and ask.

Nor is canola oil always what it seems either. Canola hydrogenates beautifully, better than corn or soybean oil, because the newer methods of hydrogenation concentrate on omega-3 fatty acids and canola is very high in omega-3s.

Since the great catering virtue of hydrogenated oils is the long shelf life and crisper texture they bring to processed foods, we would all be wise to avoid cakes and biscuits that promise to keep for months.

At most takeaway outlets, we really have no information to make our choices. There are a few worthy exceptions such as Pret a Manger who can provide information. That is why we must ask persistently and demand that answers are available to us. Surely it is not unreasonable for us to know what we're eating and what we are giving our children to eat?

In the UK, campaigners are pushing the government to act and a move towards legal regulation now seems more imminent.

Trans fats in the USA

The American market place has become increasingly aware of trans fats since a lawsuit enacted against Kraft Foods in May 2003. British-born public interest lawyer, Stephen Joseph, took the action through his lobbying organization, Ban Trans fats (www.bantransfats.com), to force Kraft to withdraw its popular Oreo cookies in California. The lawsuit asserted that the trans fat content in Oreos made them dangerous for children to eat.

According to the manufacturers, the company has sold more than 450 billion Oreo cookies since they first came onto the market in 1912.

In fact, Joseph dropped the lawsuit. He did not need to take

Kraft to court to get the trans fat issue up the agenda. He wanted to get the word out about the dangers of unlabelled trans fats in the chocolate sandwich biscuits with a cream filling. And this he did – very successfully.

This action won worldwide attention and is a classic example of how it is possible to bring about changes in the food industry through lobbying activity. Kraft Foods may not have liked the publicity but the lobbying pressured the company to create a trans fat-free Oreo cookie. It also caught the attention of influential bodies like the National Academy of Sciences' Institute of Medicine and the US Food and Drug Administration who have since taken more decisive action.

In May 2004, the Center for Science in the Public Interest (CSPI) formally petitioned the American Food and Drug Administration (FDA) to prohibit the use of HVOs in food. CSPI's Executive Director, Michael F Jacobson, says: 'Food-processing companies should worry less about the shelf-life of their products and more about the shelf-life of their customers. Getting rid of partially hydrogenated vegetable oil is probably the single easiest, fastest, cheapest way to save tens of thousands of lives each year'.

More recently, in January 2007, New York became the first city in the US to outlaw trans fats from restaurants. The city where the vast number of eating choices is so much a part of the culture has had to get rid of all but tiny traces of trans fat in its 24,000 outlets. Mayor Michael Bloomberg passed the law which forces every restaurant, café and street stall to minimize the use of trans fat to half a gram in any one item sold. Given that up until this point, an average American serving of french fries contained at least 8 grams of trans fat, this is clearly good news for the health of New Yorkers.

The action was condemned by the New York State Restaurant Association that represents some 3,500 city restaurants. The group vice president, Charles Hunt, said that compared with smoking which made other people passive victims, trans fat consumption was a matter of personal choice. He did not elaborate on how customers could assert their personal choice when they were unaware that trans fats were on the menu.

Philadelphia has followed with a similar ban and other American cities are likely to take similar action, almost certainly as a result of lobbying pressure rather than on their own initiative.

Labelling of trans fats on pre-packaged food products is already statutory in the US. However, new concerns are arising about foods sold as 'trans fat-free' when in fact they may not be. The legislation allows manufacturers to discount trans fat where the amount is less than half a gram per serving.

While chains like McDonald's, Wendy's and KFC have said they are looking for ways to cut down on the use of trans fats, a reality where none are being used is still a long way off.

Trans fats in the European Union

The truth is that the European Food Safety Authority (EFSA) has done a lot of what Europe is particularly good at: examined and reported on the issues. What it has not done is instigate any change beyond saying, 'the effect of trans fatty acids on heart health may be greater than that of saturated fatty acids'. We already knew that. We did not need its Scientific Panel on Dietetic Products, Nutrition and Allergies (NDA) to tell us this in January 2007.

The panel concluded that links to cancer, type II diabetes or allergies were 'weak or inconsistent' in spite of the vast array of clinical evidence to the contrary.

What the FSA has to date singularly failed to do is recognise the importance of shedding these superfluous, useless fats from our diet. The panel said that we consume more saturated fat than trans fat and therefore we should concentrate upon reducing saturates, but this approach ignores the fact that gram-for-gram, trans fat is far more dangerous than saturated fat.

Whether because of anxieties about how the food industry would react or just because of too much bureaucratic red tape, the reality is that Europe has done nothing to make food safer with regard to trans fat content.

Even the FSA had to acknowledge that the Mediterranean countries, where trans fat intake is the lowest in Europe, have lower levels of coronary heart disease than other member countries but it refuses to draw any conclusions.

The largest concession came from Professor Albert Flynn, Chairman of EFSA's NDA panel, who said that: 'Evidence from human intervention trials, strengthened by findings from epidemiological studies, supports the idea that the effect of trans fatty acids on heart health may be greater than that of saturated fats. However, given current intake levels of TFAs, their potential to significantly increase cardiovascular risk is much lower than that of saturates which are currently consumed in excess of dietary recommendations in many European countries'.

The report also recognized that even in the southern European countries where TFA intake was lowest, it exceeded the 10 per cent of total fat recommended as safe, and that in countries where intake is higher (including the UK), the percentage may be up to 18 per cent, almost double the accepted level.

Under current European law, hydrogenated and partially hydrogenated vegetable oils must be listed on the ingredients label but not on the nutrition label.

Trans fats in Denmark

So far, Denmark is the only country in the world to have really grasped the significance of trans fats and the potential lives to be saved by removing them. It introduced laws that regulate the sale of many foods containing trans fats. In March 2003, Denmark decided that the health of its people was more important than the short-term health of its food industry. By 1 January 2004, there was virtually no trans fat in any food item sold in the country, whether off supermarket shelves or in bars or restaurants.

As a result, Denmark is the only country in which it is possible to eat well below the one gram a day of trans fat most other countries consider to be safe, and to do so even when eating a diet largely made up of processed or ready-made food.

It all came about as a result of some initial research back in 1993 when Danish nutrition expert Walther Willet published the first studies on trans fat in *The Lancet*, demonstrating a positive association between the intake of trans fatty acids and the risk of coronary heart disease.[8]

Willet's work led to the creation of a working group to look much more closely at the whole question of trans fat in the Danish diet. A prominent cardiologist, Dr Steen Stender, was appointed as its chairman: 'The media paid a lot of attention to the presence of killer fat in food so a lot of Danes knew that it was a health hazard as early as 1994', Dr Stender recalls. 'The Danish Nutrition Council, (DNC), established in 1992, called an emergency meeting to discuss the implications [of Willett's findings]. The meeting was reported with headlines such as 'Emergency meeting on margarine hazard'. At the meeting, the council decided that the health effects of TFA deserved a thorough review and a working group was formed to fulfil that goal. Dr Stender remained in post until after the ban was fully in place.

But the initial stage in convincing both government and the public that trans fats represented a real health risk was not without its frustrations. The margarine industry reacted initially by announcing that it would be too expensive to produce margarines free of industrially produced trans fatty acids (IP-TFA) and a Swedish study group dismissed the idea that trans fats were more dangerous than saturated fats.

But as the evidence mounted, the industry began to cut back on trans fat usage and competition led to the production of zero-trans fat margarines. Many experts disagreed with the DNC's conclusions but the dairy industry was happy to see butter sales rising by 10 per cent.

'The second and third reports on TFA by the DNC were released in 2001 and 2003[9]. They found that the evidence on the harmful effects of IP-TFA, especially with regard to CHD (coronary heart disease), had been strengthened since 1994. In particular, a meta-analysis showed that an intake of approximately

8 WC Willet, MJ Stampfer et al. Intake of trans fatty acids and risk of coronary heart disease among women. *The Lancet* 1993

9 Steen Stender, Jorn Dyerberg: The influence of trans fatty acids on health, 4th edition.

5g per day of TFA was associated with a 25 per cent increased risk of CHD[10], Dr Stender explains.

This finding caught attention. It meant that gram-for-gram, trans fats were four or five times more dangerous than saturated fats. While most Danes probably weren't consuming more than a couple of grams of trans fat a day, there was the distinct possibility that some people – maybe no more than one per cent – were consuming upwards of 20 or 30g. Those with a particular fondness for foods such as french fries, biscuits and cookies, microwave popcorn and chicken nuggets would readily have consumed ten times the national average.

In Denmark in 2001, one per cent equated to 50,000 people. The UK diet will have been similar and probably heavier in its trans fat content, so for the UK at that time, there could well have been upwards of 650,000 people eating enough trans fats to increase their risk of heart disease by 150 per cent if we expostulate from the 5g/25 per cent increase equation. Unlike Denmark, we are still eating the same diet as we were seven years ago.

Dr Stender believes that there are two reasons behind Denmark's success in initiating a ban where the UK and the EU have so far failed – first of all, the weight and conviction of the Danish Nutrition Council's research, and secondly the two female politicians who spied a vote-winner through a ban. First was Ritt Bjerregaard, then finalising the legislation was Marian Fisher Boel, currently an EU commissioner.

'I hope that she has not forgotten the arguments for legislative limits', adds Dr Stender. 'An important argument for avoiding mandatory labelling is that it requires continuous public information campaigns. I certainly hope that the 500 million people in the EU need not have to learn this strange word, 'trans fat', and that the EU will adopt the Danish strategy with a legislative ban'.

In spite of the frequently voiced complaint from the food

10 CM Oomen et al: Association between trans fatty acid intake and 10-year risk of coronary heart disease in the Zutphen Elderly Study; a prospective population-based study. *Lancet* 2001

industry that HVOs are impossible to replace without compromising flavour and texture, Denmark has managed to comply with the ban and has developed trans fat-free alternatives in conjunction with the oil refining industry.

In fact, the industry complied virtually without question. Perhaps the combined assault from the scientists and the media was just too much for them to resist. By the time the Danish ban actually came into effect, most people were aware of the dangers of trans fat although Dr Stender thinks they were not necessarily particularly aware of the ban. That, he says, doesn't matter. What counts is that Danes now eat a trans fat-free diet. Everyone in the EU should be doing the same, he argues, and he is about to embark upon a mission towards making that outcome a reality.

Dorothe Pederson is Chief Consultant at the Confederation of Danish Industries. Her view is that although there was initial resistance to the ban, the industry has got over it: 'When discussions started many years ago, the industry was sceptical and reluctant to reformulate products. Trans fatty acids do have certain functionalities that are difficult to replace. As discussions went on, the industry decided that if trans fat is so harmful, it should not be in food. Today, the industry lives quite well with the Danish regulation and regards it as an advantage to have removed the trans fat.'

A Danish expert representing the confectionery industry at the time of the ban said that in fact replacing trans fats 'turned out not to be that difficult after all'. Astrid Bork Andersen and many of her colleagues would like to see an EU-wide ban that would create a level playing field and spread any additional cost in changed production techniques across all member countries.

In general, Danish experts and the Danish food industry are now aligned in their view that only a total ban throughout the EU will bring the desired effect. 'Trans fat is dispensable and is not good for public health, so let's get rid of it throughout Europe. In fact, the oil industry came up with good alternatives quite rapidly and since that development has now taken place, it shouldn't be that big a deal to implement a ban', Ms Bork Andersen believes.

Steen Stender, who led the research that ultimately brought

about the Danish ban, says the country has seen a 50 per cent fall in deaths from heart disease in the last 30 years. Not all of this can be attributed to banning trans fats in 2003, but the 20 per cent fall just since the ban was introduced does indicate a cause and effect syndrome: 'The harmful effect of industrially produced trans fat on heart disease is so well founded that the food producers using IP-TFA, in my opinion, should have the burden of proving that this is safe before they use it in the foods. In Denmark, nobody can tell a difference in taste, even with what you call the Danish pastry'.

Trans fats and Canada

Canada is one of the world's greatest consumers of trans fats. The country's administration woke up to the threat after Denmark introduced its ban. Canada passed a moderated ban through its House of Commons by an overwhelming 193-73 vote at the end of 2004.

Since December 2005, Health Canada has required that food labels list the amount of trans fat in the nutrition facts section for most foods. Like the US but with a tighter limit, products with less than 0.2g (as against 0.5g in the US) per serving are considered to be free of trans fats. The labelling includes naturally occurring trans fats as well as HVOs.

A task force was set up to implement the new requirements, and reduce the amount of trans fats in the Canadian diet. Health Canada worked along with the Heart and Stroke Foundation of Canada and recommended a limit of no more than 5 per cent of fats consumed coming from trans fat sources. The restriction meant most of the industrially produced trans fats would be removed from the Canadian diet, and about half of the remaining intake would be from naturally occurring sources (see page 13).

The recommendation has been endorsed by the Canadian Restaurants and Foodservices Association. The report's authors claim that enforcement would bring a clear and positive impact upon the health of Canadians.

But 18 months after its release, there seems to be no action by government to implement the report although the authors have lobbied it 'to act immediately on the task force's recommendations and to eliminate harmful trans fat from Canada's food supply'.

The Food & Consumer Products of Canada (FCPC) is the largest industry association representing Canadian-operated food and consumer product companies. It claims to be committed to a voluntary code that will see trans fats removed within two years.

The Canadian Heart and Stroke Foundation is disappointed by the lack of action. Its chief, Sally Brown, who co-chaired the task force of scientists, health experts and the food and restaurant industries, says: 'Trans fats are not a choice. They're a killer.' She would like to see a total ban on their use. Voluntary codes alone are difficult and slow to impact upon public health.

Lobbying for change

In spite of laudable efforts to inform and educate the public about trans fats, Europe in general, and the UK specifically, has singularly failed to take any meaningful action. While people like Dr Mary Enig, Stephen Joseph and Oliver Tickell strive to bring trans fats to the attention of health departments and the media, the powers of officialdom are disinclined to demand change. They prefer to leave the food industry to self-regulate.

Only Denmark has had the courage and tenacity to face down the food industry and put the health of its people first. Every other country in the world, where they have taken any action at all, has done so only in a very limited way and with minimal impact. If something like 275 lives could be saved *per day* in the United States alone – and that is what the research indicates – then why aren't we acting?

Perhaps previous experience has made us cynical and suspicious of simple moves that could dramatically alter our health. The tobacco industry knew for a long time before it admitted publicly that smoking was dangerous. We heard objections that a ban on smoking in public places would infringe people's inalienable human rights. We were told that we should retain the choice over whether or not to smoke and not be instructed by the 'nanny state'.

Yet, following on first from Ireland's ban on smoking on public premises, then Scotland, and in July 2007, England and Wales, people are revelling in the clean atmosphere in bars and clubs. Our clothes don't smell, our eyes don't run, and none of us has to endure the blast of smoke across a plate of food. The fears of bar proprietors' that customers would be deterred have turned out to be groundless. On the contrary, more people are going into bars than ever before because they no longer have to endure the wall of smoke. We wonder why we ever put up with it in the past. We have already almost forgotten what it was like in a bar before the ban.

Making smoking into a socially unacceptable occupation indulged in by a minority has shifted an entire cultural more within a few years. Fewer people will develop lung cancer and emphysema or its associated bronchial tract problems. More of us can breathe easily and enjoy the benefits of cleaner air at work, at leisure and when we're eating out.

We can take the lessons on board or we can ignore it and continue to be poisoned. We don't have to be. We are consumers. We buy food from supermarkets, coffee shops, sandwich shops, fast food burger outlets and other take-aways. We have the power of decision-making. All we need is a little awareness and a determination not to be put off by false claims and an industry that is far more interested in its profits than in our health and wellbeing.

What individuals can do to lobby for change:

As a consumer and a voting member of society, there is much you can do to help initiate change:

• Write to your Member of Parliament, Member of the Scottish Parliament, or Member of the Welsh or Northern Ireland Assemblies making clear your objections to the unnecessary use of trans fats in the commercial food preparation sector.

- If you have children who eat at school, make a positive effort to check the nutritional value of the food they consume. If there are trans fats present (probably in partially hydrogenated vegetable oil used for frying and in baked goods), then pressure for change.
- Ask questions at your local take-away bar. If you have a regular sandwich or coffee shop, ask them what oils and fats they use. Tell them that if they don't stop using hydrogenated vegetable oil, then you will shop elsewhere.
- Don't let your upmarket restaurant off either. Just because it has an expensive price tag and a good reputation doesn't mean it is trans fat free. Ask the chef and find out what fats are used to deep fry, bake and cook with.
- Be difficult at the in-store bakery. While some of the supermarket chains have removed trans fats from these products, the rest will comply only if pressure continues. Ask about the cookies, Danish pastries, cakes, buns, breads and muffins. You have a right to know what you and your family are eating.
- Don't delude yourself into thinking that because a chain fast food restaurant or shop has a familiar brand, the ingredients will all be safe. If you visit these kinds of outlets, ask the question: do you use hydrogenated vegetable oils anywhere in your cooking? The more of us walk away from a positive reply, the sooner we'll see change.
- Shop carefully. Yes, reading labels takes time but you will soon develop a sharp sense of where the trans fats lurk. Besides, if you thought those foods might contain, say, arsenic, you would want to ensure your choices were safe. Trans fats are just a different kind of poison.
- Cook from scratch. Wherever you can manage it, do your own cooking and do not trust to the catering and food preparation industry to do it for you. You can only know exactly what ingredients are in the dishes you prepare yourself.
- Demand quality. Why should you tolerate additives you don't feel happy with? The food retail industry will soon respond if enough of us make our voices heard.

Trans fats in the media

The media, in all its guises, creates all of our channels for the giving and receiving of information. Whether it's the winning lottery numbers, the football scores, or the news headlines, we all look to the media for information even if we rarely buy a newspaper these days. Whether it's online, via satellite, on television and radio, magazines, or through the mass of information that hits us every day from billboards, freesheets and advertising mail, we are inundated every hour of every day with it.

The media 'holds a mirror up to nature', at least in the sense that each outlet will always run with the stories that capture the interest of its readers. News and information about health and wellbeing is well up the agenda for many publications both in print copy and online. News about 'big business' conning or deluding the general public is always a powerful story and one that wins attention. Being 'poisoned' by food additives is a theme that recurs frequently. If we, as consumers, know the facts then we can reject misinformation and strive to encourage the food industry to clean up its corporate act. Perhaps this is why the issue of eating candle wax has not really caught the attention of the UK media yet. Incredibly, it is only in the last couple of years that trans fats have even started to hit the broader media agenda. Since we were unaware that there was an issue, we were not equipped to demand change. The difficulty with holding a mirror up to nature is that it has to have something to reflect upon.

This is a consumer issue on which the USA has led, Denmark has picked up the baton, and most of Europe has stayed remarkably silent. As a result, although we have benefitted to an extent from trans-Atlantic coverage, we are well behind in terms of getting trans fats out of our diet and especially out of our supermarkets and restaurants.

The campaigners

The American campaign www.bantransfats.com was founded by Stephen Joseph, the British-born lawyer who brought the landmark lawsuit against Kraft Foods on the Oreo cookie in 2003. He also led the class-action against McDonald's which ultimately brought a $7m donation from the chain as admission of its failure to follow through on the commitment to cut trans fats in its cooking oil. The climate was right. The timing was right. Government, the media, the food and catering industry could no longer ignore the issue, especially with the unequivocal medical evidence backing it: the removal of trans fats from the American diet could save at least 30,000 and maybe as many as 100,000 lives every year.

In the UK, Oliver Tickell founded www.tfx.org.uk and set about lobbying government and the public at large to push trans fats up the public health agenda. Working independently but towards the same ultimate end, these two websites have probably done more than anything or anyone else to force the food industry to begin to take action. Tickell's feature in *The Daily Express* in July 2004 was one of the first to set out the dangers in an easy-to-understand way. It was aptly headed *Face the Fats*.

A tale of two scones

One of the best in-depth reports appeared in *The Guardian* on 27 September 2006[11]. Its author, Alex Renton, has written eloquently and extensively on a range of subjects including poverty, development, food policy and food culture across the world. He describes a tasting competition between a Cookeen-based scone and a butter-based one. He watched them being prepared and baked alongside one another at Edinburgh's popular artisan bakery, the Manna House: 'When the scones emerge from the oven after 15 minutes, the vegetable fat scone is a clear winner on looks. It's gold and brown on top, with that classic toppled look, aching to be filled with cream and strawberry jam . . . the butter scones look rather squat. But when it comes to the taste test there is no contest. The butter scone melts on the tongue. It crumbles.

11 Alex Renton, Grease is the Word, The Guardian, http://environment.guardian. co.uk/print/0,,329586693-121570,00.html

It's sweet and nutty. The Cookeen scone is sort of rubbery when broken and the taste is metallic, a tap-water flavour: if I hadn't watched the process I would swear it was made with different flour'.

Renton describes a block of hydrogenated vegetable fat: 'tacky to the touch, grey-white and translucent – like the skin on a corpse', yet he recognises that it can be presented in a way that transforms it. Cookeen has since reformulated its product to remove the trans fats.

This story explains exactly why HVOs have been popular for so long. They are the commercial baker's ultimate product: cheap, easily available, keeps for months (even years), stays moist, adds good mouth-feel, and doesn't introduce any undesirable flavours. So long as the industry stayed silent on any potential health concerns, the patent secured by Proctor & Gamble in 1911 could go on producing deliciously moist delights from the deep-fryer to the grave, no problem. Alex Renton refers to a Chicago nutritionist 'who goes on television with a 22-year-old cupcake that still looks as fresh as the day it was baked'.

We have a nostalgic affection for the idea of tradition that manufacturers have no scruples about exploiting. If it's been around for a lifetime or two, then it must be good, mustn't it? The original Crisco product played on this idea remorselessly until it was forced by media coverage and clinical evidence to reformulate itself. Similarly, Oreo cookies had been around so long in America's supermarkets that they had a secure position in the minds of shoppers – until public attention revealed that they were not quite what they seemed.

How the media can help

We need the media to help us keep trans fats on the public health agenda until they are completely banished and can harm us no more. It would be easy to argue that, once armed with information, consumers can make their own decision about what products they buy or don't buy. The reality is, as is so often the case, it is those who are most vulnerable who have least choice.

Heart disease throughout the world has an alignment with poverty and deprivation. Those with the least money also have the least choice. Theirs are the diets most influenced by the cheapness of the products and the ease of access to purchase points so these people tend to be the greatest consumers of foods high in trans fats. They have neither the time nor the motivation to get out with their magnifying glasses and calculators in the Saturday afternoon check-out queues as they try to keep the kids in order and keep the shopping within a tight budget.

How supermarkets and manufacturers can help

Under pressure, British supermarkets and food manufacturers are beginning to shift from an apparently entrenched position. They are at least researching substitutes. As technological advances are made, the practical issues that previously held back the change become less significant. New oils made with a process called *interesterification* have eliminated trans fatty acids without any extra cost and even manage to keep that 'mouth-feel' the industry is so attached to. The name comes about because the component fatty acids in the oils are combined with other organic groups and are technically esters; these are shifted about within the oil molecules during the reaction.

There is already some concern among nutritionists, though, that this process may not be much better for our health than hydrogenation. The jury is still out. All the same, Denmark managed to make the switch without any big problems in 2003. Surely it cannot be beyond the imagination of UK food suppliers to do the same five years later? Can it be that the thought of using naturally-based products is so unthinkable to them as to be prohibitive?

To an extent, the good news is that trans fats are already becoming history. The food preparation and catering industries have started to divest themselves of this sticky, clinging, whitish-grey tacky block of hydrogenated vegetable oil. This is excellent news but it is certainly not the end of our problems. Trans fats continue to lurk in many of our daily foods and most of the time we still don't know they are there.

While many of the major high street supermarket chains have already committed to the removal of trans fats from their own-name lines, there is no single driver that would force the entire food production business to take hydrogenated and partially hydrogenated vegetable oil out of everything they produce. As Denmark has so clearly shown, only a legal ban could do that.

Marks & Spencer, Waitrose, Sainsbury's and Tesco say they have already removed the dangerous fats from most or all of their own lines. Asda says it is 'very nearly there' while Boots, Morrisons, Iceland and Somerfield have all confirmed that they are phasing trans fats out of their own-brand lines.

But all of this industrial action, good though it is, will impact upon only a small proportion of what we eat. Much of the food we buy in supermarkets is sold under a brand name. Mr Kipling, for example, was still producing cakes that include HVOs in November 2007 and is selling them in Sainsbury's, Tesco, Asda and many other retailers. The company has now started to reformulate its products as a result of growing awareness of the dangers and consumer-led campaigning. As long as restaurants, take-aways, in-store bakeries, commercial bakeries, confectioners and fish and chips shops are able to continue using HVOs, they will.

While they are legally entitled to produce foodstuffs that contain trans fats and not even tell us, the manufacturers are safe from attack. Our means to put them under essential pressure is to lobby through the media, getting our MPs to put up questions in parliament and through direct approaches to the manufacturers themselves. These are the techniques that, collectively, will bring the changes we want and deserve.

What labels can do to help

In the hundreds of foods we buy from take-aways and sandwich shops, we have no information about trans fat content. When we go out for a meal, whether in a modest sandwich shop or an upmarket restaurant, we don't know how much trans fat we're consuming.

Even when we're diligent with our magnifying glasses, we cannot get the whole story. There are many words and phrases for trans fats in disguise, including:

- Margarine
- Vegetable suet
- Vegetable oil solids
- Hydrogenated fat
- HVO
- PHVO

Yet the position is better than it was. Where hydrogenated or partially hydrogenated oils have been used in a pre-packaged food item, the ingredients list must declare it. This is in a way rather discriminatory because, for example, it forces the big high street bread makers like Kingsmill, Hovis, Warburton's, etc., to include HVOs in the ingredients, but the same rule doesn't apply to the French baguettes or floury bran loaves you buy from the in-store bakery. They don't have to declare anything. Mr Kipling has to declare the HVOs used in its boxed cakes, but the same is not true of the in-store bakery cookies or the coffee shop muffins.

Then there's nutrition labelling.

Surely it's not so much to ask that consumers should have food labels that give them the information they need to have in a way that is straightforward to understand? We know there is a need to control our food intake of fats, starches, proteins and minerals. We need to be able to access the information that allows us to do that.

More than half of the UK population is now overweight or obese. Most people recognise that a plate of deep-fried chips is more harmful than a baked potato, even if we were unaware of the additional danger of trans fats in deep-fried foods. The reason we do not live our lives according to that knowledge is partly because of confusing labelling and partly because we have not really taken on board the basics of how what goes in must come out. If it is not coming out through the digestive system in the normal way, then it goes into cold storage as fat that may, in turn, be lining our coronary arteries. What it cannot do is miraculously disappear.

Labels need to do a straightforward job in a straightforward way: they should tell us calories per portion and/or per pack; carbohydrate grams; the percentage of fat and whether this is saturated, unsaturated or *trans*; how much salt and sugar has been added; and the glycaemic index value.

What you can do to help

What labelling does not do now and probably never will be able to do is to give us the basics of how to eat healthily. Labels are the preserve, on the whole, of processed, ready-to-heat or ready-to-serve foods. Labels belong to instant microwave meals or frozen goods that are harmless once in a while but as a regular diet are destroying our human health.

It is this uncomfortable fact that we need to take on board. We can blame the red, amber, green lights and point out how trans fats are not included anyway, but ultimately we must decide for ourselves how we want to treat our bodies. The responsibility for our own health and wellbeing lies with our own choices although it would certainly be easier to make good choices if we were given clearer and more honest information.

CHAPTER 7

KNOW YOUR FOOD ADDITIVES

A closer examination of labels on the foods we buy will not only make us more aware of trans fats but also of some of the other undesirable ingredients lurking. Is it really necessary to add so many E-numbered flavourings and colourings, preservatives and unidentifiable substances to our food?

For the most part, these substances lengthen the shelf life of products and are added for the sake of appearance. Whether it's the red dyes added to meat to give it a 'fresh' appearance, or the bright blues and yellows of confectionery, we have learned to accept additives that have absolutely no nutritional merit of any kind.

Trans fat is not the only poison hidden away on the supermarket shelves. There are a range of other criminals, some of them perfectly fine when they form only a small part of our daily diet but are positively dangerous in larger amounts: added salt, sugar, monosodium glutamate, flavourings, colourings, and preservatives, for example. For certain vulnerable groups, such as children or those with asthma, some of these are dangerous even in small amounts.

Here are some of the most frequently used additives you will find on food labels, and a description of what they are. I also note the generally agreed consensus on the safety or otherwise of the additives, but remember, new research is being carried out all the time – today's 'safe' could be tomorrow's 'suspect'.

The major E-numbers

E100 Curcumin Orange-yellow colouring from the root of the curcuma (turmeric) plant. Used as a preservative, colourant and flavouring agent in many food products including baked foods, pickles and meat products. An essential ingredient in many Indian dishes, turmeric aids digestion and may have some medical benefits. Along with Annatto (E160b), it is also used to colour cheeses, dry mixes, salad dressings, winter butter and margarine, and is dissolved in alcohol for water-containing products such as pickles, relishes and mustard.
Possible side effects Safe in recommended doses but best avoided by people with gallstones, obstructive jaundice, acute bilious colic, or toxic liver disorders.

E101 and E101a Riboflavin Yellow or orange-yellow colouring used to fortify some foods, especially baby foods, breakfast cereals, sauces, processed cheese, fruit drinks and vitamin-enriched milk products as well as in vitamin supplements.
Possible side effects None known, but it will almost certainly be the result of genetic modification.

E102 Tartrazine A synthetic yellow dye used in fruit drinks and coloured fizzy drinks, instant puddings, cake mixes, custard powder, soups, sauces, ice cream, ice pops, sweets, chewing gum, marzipan, jam, jelly, marmalade, mustard, yoghurt and many more convenience foods. It is also used to make the shells of medicinal capsules. Banned in Norway and Austria but widely used in the UK.
Possible side effects Best avoided for children following some evidence of a link with ADHD. It can also cause allergies in asthmatics and those with an aspirin intolerance. Reactions have included migraine, blurred vision, itching, rhinitis and purple skin patches.

E104 Quinoline Yellow Colouring, often called the synthetic 'coal tar' dye, present in ice cream, scotch eggs and smoked haddock. Also in lipsticks, hair products, colognes and medications. Banned in Australia, Japan, Norway and the United States.

Possible side effects May cause dermatitis and should certainly be avoided for children, as it can increase hyperactivity.

Azo dyes

Azo dyes account for about 60-70 per cent of all the dyes used in food and textile manufacture and practically every colour can be produced simply and cheaply using them.

Possible side effects Our bodies don't retain azo colourants. A human being would need to eat about 100kg of azo-coloured food in a day to consume a dangerous dose. All the same, some azo dyes have been banned for food use not because of the dyes themselves but because of the way in which some of them break down in the human body. ADHD in children has often been linked to these food dyes but research remains inconsistent. It seems most likely that a combination of azo dyes and benzoic acid may be a trigger for sensitive children.

E110 Sunset Yellow/Orange Yellow Like E104, this is an azo or synthetic coal tar dye present especially in fermented foods. You will find it in all the same products as E102 and E104 but also in Swiss rolls, lemon curd, hot chocolate mix, breadcrumb coating, cheese sauce and canned fish. Banned in Norway and Finland but widely used in the UK.

Possible side effects This is one worth avoiding, especially for children and those with an aspirin intolerance. It has been shown to cause hives, rhinitis, nasal congestion, hyperactivity, abdominal pain, nausea and vomiting, indigestion and a distaste for food. More seriously, it is associated with kidney tumours and chromosomal damage. Research has shown an increased incidence of tumours in animals given E110.

E120 Cochineal, Carmic Acid, Carmines An expensive red colouring, not suitable for vegetarians as it is extracted from the crushed carcasses of the female *Dactylopius coccus*, a cactus-feeding scale insect, which are killed by either immersion in hot water or by exposure to sunlight, steam or the heat of an oven. The variety in the appearance of commercial cochineal is caused by these differing extraction methods. Found in alcoholic drinks, bakery products and toppings, biscuits, desserts, drinks, icings, pie fillings, some varieties of cheddar cheese, sauces and sweets.
Possible side effects May cause allergic reactions. Not recommended for consumption by children where it may increase hyperactivity.

E122 Carmoisine/Azorubine A synthetic red azo dye used in foods that need to be heat-treated following fermentation and also found in blancmange, marzipan, Swiss roll, jams and preserves, confectionery, brown sauce, flavoured yogurts, packet soups, jellies, breadcrumb coating and cheesecake mixes. Banned in Japan, Norway, Sweden and the United States but in common use in the UK.
Possible side effects Again, not suitable for children because it may increase hyperactivity levels. Also avoid if you have asthma or a sensitivity to aspirin.

E123 Amaranth A purplish-red or blackcurrant synthetic coal tar or azo dye common in ice cream, gravy granules, jams, jelly, tinned fruit pie fillings, prawns, packet cake mix, soups and trifles. Although derived originally from the small herbaceous plant of the same name, amaranth has developed a mixed press. It is banned in Norway, the United States, Russia and Austria with a very restricted use in France and Italy.
Possible side effects Some research shows amaranth to provoke asthma, eczema and hyperactivity. It also caused birth defects and foetal deaths in some animal tests.

E124 Ponceau 4R/Cochineal Red A/Brilliant Scarlet 4R A red synthetic coal tar or azo dye found in dessert toppings, jelly, salami, seafood dressings, tinned strawberries and fruit pie fillings, packet cake mixes, cheesecakes, soups and trifles. Banned in Norway and the United States.

Possible side effects Seems to cause allergic and/or intolerance reactions particularly among those with an aspirin intolerance or asthmatics, and increases hyperactivity and behavioural disorders in children. Carcinogenic in animals.

E127 Erythrosine You are most likely to meet E127 in dental disclosing tablets but this cherry pink/red synthetic coal tar dye is also found in many kinds of pre-packaged processed cherries, in canned fruit, custard mix, sweets, bakery, snack foods, biscuits, chocolate, dressed crab, garlic sausage, luncheon meat, salmon spread, pâté, scotch eggs, stuffed olives and packet trifle mix. Banned in Norway and the United States.

Possible side effects May cause an increase in thyroid activity and it was shown to cause thyroid cancer in rats in a study. There may be a link with hyperactivity. Best avoided for children.

E128 Red 2G The UK is the only EU country still using Red 2G. It is also banned in Australia, Austria, Canada, Japan, Norway, Sweden and the United States. A red synthetic coal tar or azo dye found mainly in cooked meat products and sausages but sometimes in jams and drinks.

Possible side effects Concerns that it can interfere with blood haemoglobin. Not recommended for consumption by children.

E129 Allura Red AC Orange-red colour used in sweets, drinks and condiments, medications and cosmetics. A red synthetic azo dye introduced in the early 1980s to replace Amaranth in the United States of America where it is prohibited. Banned in Denmark, Belgium, France, Germany, Switzerland, Sweden, Austria and Norway.

Possible side effects May have slightly reduced tolerance for asthmatics and aspirin-intolerant individuals. Association with skin sensitivity and cancer in mice. Avoid for children.

E131 Patent Blue V A dark bluish-violet synthetic coal tar dye that is not very widely used now but still crops up occasionally in

Scotch eggs. Banned in Australia, the United States and Norway.
Possible side effects Can cause skin reaction with itching and
nausea, low blood pressure, tremors and breathing problems.
Avoid for children.

E132 Indigo Carmine/Indigotine Blue synthetic coal tar dye in
use since 1890 when the Prussian research chemist, Adolf von
Baeyer worked out the chemical structure of indigo. It is produced by a synthesis of indoxyl by fusion of sodium
phenylglycinate in a mixture of caustic soda and sodamide. Used
in tablets and capsules as well as ice cream, sweets and baked
goods.
Possible side effects Can cause skin reaction with itching and
nausea, low blood pressure, tremors and breathing problems.
Avoid for children.

E133 Brilliant Blue Often used along with Tartrazine E102 to
produce a whole range of blue-green shades, it is found in tinned
processed peas, some dairy products, ice cream, confectionery
and soft drinks as well as soaps and shampoo. Banned in Austria,
Belgium, Denmark, France, Germany, Greece, Italy, Norway,
Spain, Sweden and Switzerland.
Possible side effects Not recommended for consumption by children because of a link with hyperactivity.

E140 Chlorophylls, Chlorophyllins Green colour that occurs naturally in the cells of all plants and is responsible for
photosynthesis. Chlorophyll is fairly unstable as a dye and fades
easily. Produced from nettles, spinach and grass using acetone
and used to dye waxes and oils in medicines and cosmetics. It is
also found in chewing gum, fats and oils, ice cream, soaps, soups,
sweets and, of course, green vegetables.
Possible side effects None known.

E141 Copper complexes of chlorophylls and cholorphyllins Olive
green soluble colour and a water-soluble green colour derived
from E140 chlorophyll by substituting copper for magnesium to
increase stability. Found in some cheeses, chewing gum, ice

cream, parsley sauce, soups and green vegetable and fruits pre-served in liquids.
Possible side effects Nothing as yet proven but some grounds for suspicion. Best avoided.

E142 Green S/Acid Brilliant Green BS A green synthetic coal tar dye found in desserts, gravy granules, ice cream, mint sauce, sweets, packet breadcrumbs, cake mixes and tinned peas. Banned in Canada, Finland, Japan, Norway, Sweden and the United States.
Possible side effects Research is ongoing into acceptable intake levels but is known to cause hyperactivity, asthma, uticaria and insomnia. Best avoided, especially for children.

Caramel colourings

E150a-E150d Caramel These colourings range from dark brown to black and are made by controlled heat treatment of sugar beet or sugar cane. This is the most widely used group of colourings and makes up 98 per cent of all the colours used in commercial production. Caramel is used widely in beer, brown bread, buns, chocolate, biscuits, brandy, chocolate-flavoured flour-based cakes, coatings, decorations, fillings and toppings, crisps, dessert mixes, doughnuts, fish and shellfish spreads, frozen desserts, glucose tablets, gravy browning, ice cream, jams, milk desserts, pancakes, pickles, sauces and dressings, soft drinks (particularly cola drinks), stouts, sweets, vinegar, whisky and wine.
Possible side effects Not recommended for consumption by children but there is really no solid evidence of any problems linked to caramel-based colourings.

E151 Brilliant Black/Black PN Brown and violet-black colourant similar to E104, used in decorations and coatings, desserts, fish paste, flavoured milk drinks, ice cream, mustard, red fruit jams, sauces, savoury snacks, soft drinks, soups and confectionery. Banned in Denmark, Australia, Austria, Belgium, Canada, Finland, France, Germany, Japan, Norway, Switzerland, Sweden, USA and Norway .

Possible side effects Best avoided for children as it may increase hyperactivity.

E153 Carbon Black/Vegetable Carbon This black colouring comes from a range of sources including activated charcoal, bones, meat, blood, various fats, oils and resins but is mostly derived from burnt vegetable matter. It may include genetically modified crops and vegetarians should be aware that it can be of animal origin. It is mostly found in concentrated fruit juices, jams, jellies and liquorice. It is banned as a food additive in the United States.

Possible side effects Suspected as a carcinogen although the link is so far unproven. Best avoided with children and anyone with a tendency towards allergies or intolerances in food.

E154 Brown FK, Kipper Brown This is a highly suspect additive that has been banned everywhere in the EU except the UK. It's also prohibited in Australia, Austria, Canada, Finland, Ireland, Japan, Norway, Sweden and the United States. You will find it mainly in kippers and smoked mackerel but occasionally also in cooked hams and crisps.

Possible side effects Has been blamed for increased aggression but the research is inconclusive. Best avoided by asthmatics.

E160a Alpha, Beta, Gamma Carotene Orange or yellow plant pigments sourced from carrots. Fades on exposure to light. Used in butter and soft margarines, coffee sponge cakes, milk products and soft drinks.

Possible side effects Very high amounts are associated with yellowing of the skin. As carotene is a source of vitamin A, high concentrations will cause symptoms of vitamin A toxicity.

E160b Annatto, Bixin, Norbixon A yellow–red vegetable dye that comes from the seed coat of the fruit of the Annatto tree, *Bixa*

orellana. This has largely taken over from Tartrazine E102, but the hyperactive child support groups think it may be as guilty as its predecessor. Sometimes used with E100 Curcumin in cheese, coleslaw, crisps, custard, fish fingers, flavoured instant mashed potato, fruit and cream fillings and toppings, frying oil, ice cream, lollies, icings, liqueurs, low-calorie spreads, margarine, meat balls, salad cream, mayonnaise, smoked fish, soft drinks, sponge cakes and puddings, steak and kidney pie, pastry and yoghurt. Also used as a body paint, digestive aid and expectorant as well as in soap, fabric dye and varnishes.
Possible side effects May cause allergies and eczema.

E160c Paprika Extract, Capsanthin, Capsorubin Orange–red colouring extracted from the fruit pod and seeds of the red pepper, *Capsicum annuum*. Used widely in poultry feed to deepen the colour of the egg yolks and can also be found in cheese slices and chicken pies. It is likely to become more frequently used as synthetic colours become less popular. Not permitted in Australia.
Possible side effects None known.

E160d Lycopene This is a red colourant extracted from tomatoes and pink grapefruit. Not in wide use. There has been some research that suggests Lycopene could have anti-cancer properties but it is not clear whether the quantities as a food additive would be appropriate. Not permitted in Australia.
Possible side effects None known.

E160e Beta-apo-8' carotenal (C30) An orange–red colouring, normally synthetic as a food colour though it occurs naturally in oranges and tangerines. Can be found in cheese slices.
Possible side effects None known.

E160f: Ethyl-ß-apo-8'-carotenate (ethyl ester of ß-apo-8'-carotenic acid) A natural orange-yellow through to dark red food colour present in many plants and made commercially out of E160e. Used in a vast range of different products.
Possible side effects None known.

E161a Flavoxanthin A natural yellow food colour commercially produced from buttercup but rarely used now – occasionally found in confectionery.
Possible side effects None known.

E161b Lutein Natural yellow, not much used, occasionally found in soups and alcoholic beverages, Lutein is commercially produced from grass, nettles or *Tagetes* species.
Possible side effects None known.

E161c Cryptoxanthin, E161d Rubixanthin, E161e Violaxanthin, E161f Rhodoanthin Natural yellow colourings, used sometimes in confectionery.
Possible side effects None known.

E161g Canthaxanthin A natural orange derived from *catharelles* (mushrooms) but most is synthetically produced from carotene. This is the main ingredient in tanning pills and is also widely used as a food colouring.
Possible side effects Often associated with eye problems when used in tanning pills but doesn't seem to have any side effects when used as a food colourant.

E162 Beetroot Red/Betanin Beetroot colouring commonly used in frozen and preserved foods. The beet (*Beta vulgaris*) is a flowering plant in the family *Amaranthaceae*.

Beetroot extract or pulp has been used to colour food for centuries, but it is only since the early 20th century that it has become commonly used as a commercially produced additive.
Possible side effects None known – but it does tend to produce intensely coloured urine!

E163a–f, i–iii Anthocyanins A large group of natural colours ranging from orange to purple that come from fruit, flowers and berries. Individual compounds are isolated from different plant species. These extracts are used in a wide variety of food and drink products.

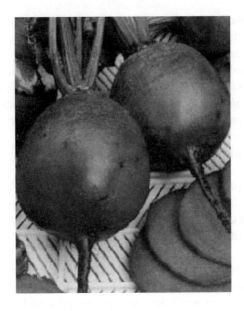

Possible side effects None known.

E171 Calcium Carbonate (chalk), E170 (i) Calcium Carbonate, E170 (ii) Calcium Hydrogen Carbonate (CI77220) An inorganic natural white mineral compound that is perfectly safe. It is used as a surface coating, an anti-caking agent, filling agent in pharmaceuticals, and a stabiliser in canned fruit.
Possible side effects None known.

E171 Titanium Dioxide Inorganic whitening agent, most familiar to us in the form of toothpaste and also used to separate the layers in products.
Possible side effects None known.

E172i–iii Iron Oxides and Hydroxides Naturally forming inorganic minerals commercially produced using iron powder which is not absorbed into the body. These oxides are used for numerous surface coatings.
Possible side effects None known.

E173 Aluminium Silver-grey colouring used only for surface coating.
Possible side effects We take in more aluminium from natural food sources than from additives. High concentrations of aluminium may cause several side effects in humans but research is inconclusive with much of it now discredited, especially regarding any linkage with Alzheimer's Disease.

E174 Silver Like Aluminium, a silver-grey colouring used (rarely) for surface coating.
Possible side effects None known.

E175 Gold Gold colouring used (rarely) for surface coating.
Possible side effects None known.

E180 Pigment Rubine/Lithol Rubine BK Synthetic azo dye (see box for more about azo dyes).

E200 Sorbic Acid, E201Sodium Sorbate, E202 Potassium Sorbate, E203 Calcium Sorbate A naturally occurring preservative that comes from the fruit of the European Mountain-ash (Sorbus aucuparia) and is commercially produced in several different chemical processes. Mainly used to protect against the growth of fungi and yeasts. Used in a wide range of products including many yoghurts and other fermented dairy products, fruit salads, confectionery, lemonade, cheese, rye bread, cakes and bakery products, pizza, shellfish, lemon juice, wine, cider and soups.
Possible side effects Generally none in the small concentrations used but there have been some individual complaints of headaches and intestinal upset.

E210 Benzoic Acid, E211 Sodium Benzoate, E21 Potassium Benzoate, E21 3Calcium Benzoate, E214 Ethyl 4-hydroxybenzoate, E215 Ethyl 4-hydroxybenzoate, E216 Propyl 4-hydroxybenzoate, E217 Propyl 4-hydroxybenzoate, E218 Methyl 4-hydroxybenzoate, E219 Methyl 4-hydroxybenzoate, Sodium Salt. All of these are synthetically produced preservatives. Naturally, benzoic acid, benzoates and benzoic acid esters are found in most fruit, especially cranberries, and in mushrooms, cinnamon, cloves and some dairy products. Commercially, the benzoates are prepared chemically from toluene, a by-product of crude oil that smells like paint thinner and has the capacity to dissolve paint, rubber, adhesives and disinfectant. Toluene is used as an octane booster in petrol and in the preparation of TNT. Benzoic acid and benzoates are used as preservatives against yeasts and bacteria in acidic products.

Possible side effects Toluene consumed in Benzoic Acid is not the same as sniffing it to get high. All the same, the association with a highly toxic, potentially brain destroying, substance is not reassuring. Our bodies are unable to secrete toluene. We have to metabolise it to get rid of it. Many parents of hyperactive children or children with behavioural problems such as aggressiveness and poor concentration are convinced of the linkage. A 2007 study carried out by Southampton University confirmed these beliefs and also a linkage with asthma and skin rashes. A theory that the combination of any of this group of benzoates with certain food colourings (*Tartrazine E102, Ponceau-4R E124, Sunset yellow E110, Allura red AC E129*) is particularly dangerous for this group of sensitive children is gathering credibility.

E220 Sulphur Dioxide Although often associated with the smell of rotten eggs, sulphur dioxide is in fact a very old and effective preservative used from ancient Egyptian times and still essential today, especially in wine-making. It acts as an antibiotic and antioxidant, protecting the wine from organisms that would otherwise cause spoilage and oxidation. So long as the concentrations are low in wine (under 350ppm), taste is not detectable. It is also used as a preservative for dried fruit where it helps retain the natural colour and as a bleaching agent in flour.

Possible side effects Can reduce the vitamin content in products but is not dangerous in normal concentrations. May irritate asthma sufferers and in high concentrations can cause gastrointestinal upset.

E221 Sodium Sulphite Similar in its function to E220 and used as a bleaching agent to prevent spoilage and discoloration. Used in bread because it improves the kneading capacity. It is found in eggs and products with egg yolk, salads, beer, bread and caramel.

Possible side effects Because of its oxidising effect, it can reduce the vitamin content in certain products. It is reduced in the liver to harmless sulphate and excreted in the urine.

E222 Sodium Metabisulphite, E223 Sodium Disulphite, E224 Potassium Disulphite, E225 Potassium Sulphite, E226 Calcium Sulphite, E227 Calcium Hydrogen Sulphite Similar to E221 these are another synthetic preservatives and bleaching agents used mainly in preserved onions, alcoholic drinks including whisky and beer, bakery products, fruit juices and a wide range of potato products. E226 is also used to increase the firmness of canned vegetables.

Possible side effects Because of its oxidising effect, it can reduce the vitamin content in certain products. It is reduced in the liver to harmless sulphate and excreted in the urine.

E230 Biphenyl, Diphenyl, Phenylbenzene, Lemonene, E231 Phenylphenol, Hydroxybiphenyl, E232 Sodium Biphenyl-2-yl oxide, E233 2-Thiazol-4-yl Benzimadazole As E210-219 this is a preservative derived from benzene. It is a solid organic compound that forms colourless to yellowish crystals. It has a distinctively pleasant aroma and is used against *Penicillium* fungi growing on citrus fruit. It is used on the containers to kill bacteria and to impregnate the wrapping on citrus fruits. Sometimes fruits are dipped in a solution of diphenyl, which slowly penetrates the peel and may be present in the fruit itself.

E234 Nisin, E235 Pimaracin, Natamycin Natural antibiotics produced by bacterium, normally used in cheese and meat production as a preservative against spoilage bacteria. Also in cream and canned fruits.

Possible side effects As it is a protein, it is treated by the body as such and digested in the small intestine.

E236 Formic Acid, Methanoic Acid This is used against a range of micro-organisms but is unpopular because of its smell. It is naturally present in ants and in many fruits such as apples, strawberries and raspberries as well as in honey and nettles. Commercially, it is produced from sulphuric acid, sodium hydroxide and carbon monoxide. Used in beverages, bakery products, sweets and ice cream.
Possible side effects At high concentrations, it has a diuretic effect, it is normally metabolised in the liver and excreted.

E237 Formic Acid Sodium Salt, Sodium Formate, E238 Calcium Formate Essentially a salt preservative the same as *E236* but made from carbon monoxide and sodium hydroxide it is used against micro-organisms in fruit juices, other non-alcoholic beverages and preserved vegetables.
Possible side effects Metabolised in the liver and excreted normally.

E239 Hexamine and E240 Formaldehyde It sounds alarming to say that hexamine is commercially synthesised from formaldehyde – traditionally used in embalming to preserve human remains – but actually formaldehyde is present in the atmosphere in tobacco smoke, smoke from forest fires and in car exhaust fumes as well as in pre-washes and toothpaste. Formaldehyde gas is not used in food preparation but can be used to disinfect containers, pipes and vessels in the industry and is widely used in cosmetics.
Possible side effects Although the EU is considering a total ban on the use of formaldehyde, including for embalming, it is probably not dangerous in the small amounts used in food preservation. Large exposure is, though, potentially lethal. Concentrations above 0.1 parts per million (ppm) in the air can cause irritation to the eyes and mucous membranes. If inhaled, formaldehyde at this concentration may cause headaches, a burning sensation in the throat, and cause difficulty breathing, as well as triggering or aggravating asthma symptoms.

E242 Dimethylcarbonate A cold sterilisation preservative in soft drinks

Possible side effects None.

E249 Potassium Nitrite, E250 Potassium Nitrate, E251 Sodium Nitrate, E252 Potassium Nitrate Naturally occurring mineral used as a preservative against *Clostridium botulinum*, a bacterium that can cause botulism, in meat and fish products.

Possible side effects Nitrites are the forerunners of possibly carcinogenic nitrosamines which are formed in the stomach from nitrites and proteins. High concentrations may react with haemoglobin in the blood. Potassium nitrite is not permitted in products intended for children under a year-old because their haemoglobin reacts much more to it than the adult form.

E260 Acetic Acid, Ethanoic Acid, E261 Potassium Acetate, E262 Sodium Acetate, E263 Calcium Acetate Used as a preservative against bacteria, especially in mayonnaise where it is used to protect against *Salmonella*, and also in fungi. It is most effective in acidic foods. Naturally present in most fruits, it is produced by bacterial fermentation, but commercially it is made in the bacterial fermentation of sugar, molasses or alcohol or by chemical synthesis from acetealdehyde.

Possible side effects Minimal risk but some sensitive individuals have complained of headaches, intestinal upset and skin disorders.

E270 Lactic Acid, E325 Sodium Lactate, E326 Potassium Lactate, E327 Calcium Lactate Naturally produced by bacteria in fermented foods and commercially by bacterial fermentation on starch and molasses, lactic acid is also produced in large amounts in the large intestine. It is used as a preservative, protecting against yeasts and fungi and to increase the stability of potato products, so it appears in a very wide range of acidic products.

Possible side effects No side effects in adults. D- or DL-lactates (stereoisomers) should not be given to babies and small children as they have not yet developed the appropriate enzymes in the liver to metabolise these forms of lactate. E270 does not contain milk.

E280 Propionic Acid, E281 Sodium Propionate, E282 Calcium Propionate, E283 Potassium Propionate Like lactic acid, propionic acid (and its salt) is already present in the large intestine and is a normal component of sweat. It is also produced by bacteria in the fermentation process for certain types of cheese. It is a preservative, mainly against fungi, and often used in bakery goods. Its strong smell limits its applications.

Possible side effects None, because it is already in many of the body's metabolic pathways.

E284 Boric Acid, E285 Sodium Tetraborate A natural acid, produced commercially from boron, used as a buffer to control acidity levels and as a mineral source in various multi-vitamin/mineral compounds, also as a mild antiseptic and to treat or prevent certain fungal infections such as athlete's foot and candida. It is also used in some eye preparations as the only acid actually beneficial to the eyes. Rarely used in food but regularly in pharmaceuticals, boric acid is also an insecticide and popular with fire eaters for the bright green flame it emits!

Possible side effects No more dangerous than table salt in low concentrations but more questionable in pharmaceuticals where concentrations can be very high.

E290 Carbon Dioxide Literally in the air we breathe. In the food industry, it is used in some pre-packed foods and to carbonate soft drinks.

Possible side effects None known from use in food.

E296 Malic Acid Natural acid present in most fruits and many vegetables, malic acid is commercially produced using chemical synthesis. It is part of the metabolic pathway of every living cell and is used as a flavour compound and colour stabiliser in apple and grape juices.

Possible side effects None known but high concentrations are not allowed in infant food since small children lack the capacity to metabolise large amounts of malic acid.

E297 Fumaric Acid A natural acid in many fruits and vegetables. Commercially made by fermentation of sugar with fungi or by chemical synthesis. It is, like malic acid, part of the metabolic pathway in all living cells. Used as the acid source in baking powder and as acid and structure stabiliser in a large range of products.

Possible side effects Nothing known.

E300 L-Ascorbic Acid (Vitamin C), E301 Sodium Ascorbate, E302 Calcium Ascorbate, E303 Potassium Ascorbate Vitamin C occurs naturally in most fruits and vegetables, especially citrus fruit. Ascorbic acid is commercially synthesised by bacterial fermentation of glucose, followed by chemical oxidation but cannot be labelled as vitamin C if it is labelled E300 because it is then functioning as an anti-oxidant rather than a vitamin supplement. A shortage of vitamin C can lead to scurvy.

Possible side effects None as a food additive. Overdose of Vitamin C can cause diarrhoea.

E304 Fatty acid esters of ascorbic acid A combination of the fatty acid palmitate with ascorbic acid (vitamin C) produced from fat. It is added to prevent rancidity in plant oils with many unsaturated fatty acids thus giving longer shelf-life where HVOs have been rejected.

Possible side effects None known in the concentrations used in food. Palmitic acid is usually obtained from vegetable fat but occasionally from animal fat, including pork, so may be unsuitable for some diets.

E306 Tocopherol concentrate, E307 Alpha-tocopherol, E308 Gamma-tocopherol, E309 Delta-tocopherol Extracted from vegetable oils rich in tocopherols (Vitamin E) and used to prevent rancidity in animal oils but as it imparts a powerful flavour, uses are limited.

Possible side effects Although high doses of vitamin E can be toxic, these levels are not reached from food additives.

E310 Propyl Gallate, E311 Octyl Gallate, E312 Dodecyl Gallate An anti-oxidant synthesised from propanol and gallic acid and used to control rancidity in many fatty products and cosmetics.

Possible side effects Gallic acid can cause eczema, stomach problems and hyperactivity.

E315 Erythorbic Acid, E316 Sodium Erythorbate Synthetic isomer of Vitamin C but with only 1/20 of the vitamin activity, this is an anti-oxidant that is similar to the plant tannin-based *E310, E311, and E312.*
Possible side effects None known in the concentrations in use.

E320 Butylated Hydroxyanisole, E321 Butylated Hydroxytoluene Synthetic anti-oxidant present in fats and fatty products to prevent rancidity.
Possible side effects May increase hyperactivity in susceptible children and those with asthma may react badly. Be cautious if you suffer from any allergies or intolerances. Best avoided for babies and infants. BHA, along with high concentrations of Vitamin C, can produce the free radicals which cause damage to the components of cells, including DNA. The EU is in the process of restricting the use of BHA.

E322 Lecithins Emulsifier that helps to stop the fat from separating out in foods. It comes mainly from high fat foods such as eggs and beef liver but is also found in peanuts, beef steak and some fruits and vegetables. There has been a surge of alternative health interest in lecithin with claims that it may improve memory, lower cholesterol and improve liver function. It contains phosphatidycholine, a phospholipid that is crucial to every cell in the body without which our cell membranes would harden up. Lecithin also protects cells from oxidation and is the main component in the protective sheath around the human brain. However, the research to date is inconsistent and a 1989 review of 24 studies published in the American Journal of Clinical Nutrition concluded that there was little evidence that lecithin directly lowers cholesterol (*Knuiman et al, 1989*).
Possible side effects Since it is a normal component of all our cells, lecithin causes no side effects and is broken down by the body and expelled with no problems. It doesn't cause allergic

reactions in people allergic to soybeans or eggs and is suitable for all diets.

E330 Citric Acid, E331 Sodium Citrates, E332 Potassium Citrates, E333 Calcium Citrates Part of the key metabolic pathways in all our body cells, citric acid is found in every living organism. Large amounts are present in many fruits, especially kiwi, strawberries and citrus fruits. It is commercially prepared by fermentation of molasses with the mould, *Aspergillus niger*. Citric acid is useful for a range of applications in food. It increases the gel strength in marmalades and cuts back on the browning of fruits cause by enzymes. It's also used as a flavour and aroma enhancer in products like orange squash.

Possible side effects Already a normal part of our body function and cell maintenance, there is not likely to be any unnatural reaction to citric acid although some reports suggest intolerances.

E334 Tartaric Acid, E335 Sodium Tartrate, E336 Potassium Tartrate, E337 Potassium Sodium Tartrate Although already present in most fruits, tartaric acid is commercially prepared from waste grape skins as a by-product of the wine-making industry. Used as an acidity regular and to stabilise colour, it also enhances fruit flavour and is found in confectionery, soft drinks, wine and marmalade.

Possible side effects As it's a natural substance, it is safely excreted in the urine with no side-effects.

E338 Orthophosphoric Acid, E339 Sodium Phosphates, E340 Potassium Phosphates, E341 Calcium Phosphates These are all variants used in slightly differing ways in different foods to regulate acidity. They increase the permeability of salt in meats, act as an anti-oxidant or an emulsifier, stop desiccation or clumping in powder products, and so appear in a wide variety of products from bread to cola, including meat and cheese products, baking powder and tooth whitening products.

Possible side effects Phosphates are a normal body salt and their use as a food additive has no side effects. Some people have been anxious about phosphates, associating them with animal bones but no bones are used in commercial production which is done from phosphate mined in the US.

E350 Sodium Malates, E351 Potassium Malate, E352 Calcium Malate A natural acid present in fruit, the malates are used as a buffer and flavouring in a variety of foods including soft drinks, confectionery, ice cream and fried products.
Possible side effects None. Best avoided for infants who are unable to metabolise certain compounds in the malates.

E353 Meta-tartaric Acid Acidity regulator present in sugar cane and produced from glucose, it is used in wine and fruit juices.
Possible side effects None known.

E354 Calcium Tartarate A natural acid in fruit, it is used as an acidity regulator and preservative in fish and fruit preserves, seaweed products and in the pharmaceuticals industry.
Possible side effects None known; it is metabolised in the body to tartaric acid.

E355 Adipic Acid, E356 Sodium Adipate, E357 Potassium Adipate Natural acid in beets and sugar cane used as an acidity regulator and aroma compound, present in a wide range of products including low-sodium and herbal salts.
Possible side effects None known; it is metabolised and excreted in urine.

E363 Succinic Acid Natural acid present in all cells and commercially produced from acetic acid (vinegar), it is used as an acidity regulator and flavour enhancer in a wide range of products.
Possible side effects None known.

E380 triAmmonium Citrate A synthetic acidity regulator, buffer and emulsifier used in chocolate confectionery, cheese spreads and other products.
Possible side effects None known. Citric acid is a normal component in body cells.

E385 *Calcium Disodium EDTA* This synthetic compound is sometimes used as a treatment for people who have suffered heavy metal intoxication because it binds to the metals and removes them from the body. Otherwise, it's in a range of products as a stabiliser.
Possible side effects None known. If taken in very high doses, it could deplete iron resources.

E400 *Alginic Acid*, E401 *Sodium Alginate*, E402 *Potassium Alginate*, E403 *Ammonium Alginate*, E404 *Calcium Alginate*, E404 *Propane-1, 2-Diol Alginate*, E406 *Agar*, E407 *Carrageenan*, E410 *Locust Bean Gum (Carob Gum)*, E412 *Guar Gum*, E413 *Tragacanth*, E414 *Gum Acacia (Gum Arabic)*, E415 *Xanthan Gum* This is the group of thickening agents and emulsifiers which all come from natural sources such as seaweed and plants and are used in a range of products including ice cream, confectionery, soft drinks, food colourings, icings, salad dressings and frozen bakery products.
Possible side effects On the whole, these additives are safe. Some may cause minor discomfort, flatulence or a bloated feeling because of fermentation in the gut, as all indigestible polysaccharides will.

E420 *Sorbitol* Natural sweetener that is present in many berries and fruits including apples, prunes, cherries and grapes. It is commercially produced from glucose (dextrose). Commercially, it is mostly used as a stabiliser, low-calorie sweetener and bulking agent. It is present in many bakery and confectionery products, especially those presented as 'diabetic'.
Possible side effects Sorbitol is partly absorbed and metabolised as fructose by the body and can raise blood sugar levels in much the same way as sucrose. Sorbitol should not be regarded by diabetics as a no-carbohydrate sweetener. It can cause diarrhoea in larger amounts (more than 20 grams) and flatulence and should not be consumed by infants under a year old.

E421 *Mannitol* Another natural sweetener. Present in many plants including conifers, seaweed and mushrooms. It is commercially

produced from glucose. It is used as an anti-caking agent, low-calorie sweetener, and bulking agent in bakery and confectionery products.
Possible side effects Can cause flatulence and bloating and may have a laxative effect in large amounts.

E422 Glycerol Like E420 and E421, a natural carbohydrate alcohol which is one of the components of all fats. It is present in low concentrations in the blood. Commercially, it can be produced synthetically from propane or by bacterial fermentation of sugars. It is used as a low-calorie sweetener and also helps keep bakery and confectionery products moist.
Possible side effects Absorbed and metabolised as glucose and converted to fat.

E440 Pectins A natural acid polysaccharide present in most fruit, it is commercially produced from apple pulp and orange peels. Pectin is used as a thickening agent, emulsifier and stabiliser in preserves, fruit jellies and sauces.
Possible side effects Sometimes used in diet products to promote a feeling of fullness that can also lead to intestinal problems.

E450 (i)-(vi) Potassium and Sodium Diphosphates; E451 Potassium and Sodium Tri-phosphates Various salts of sodium/potassium/calcium with phosphates that are synthetically produced from the respective carbonates and phosphoric acid. These have a whole range of food uses as buffers and emulsifiers and can even bind metals.
Possible side effects None known in food use.

E452 (i)-(v) Polyphosphates Similar to E450 above but also used to retain water during processing and storage.
Possible side effects None known in food use.

E460 Cellulose, E461 Methylcellulose, E463 Hydroxpropyl-cellulose, E464 Hydroxpropyl-Methylcellulose, E465 Ethyl-methylcellulose, E466 Carboxymethylcellulose Cellulose comes from wood and some plants and is mainly used as a thickening agent, a filler, for dietary fibre, as an anti-clumping agent and as an emulsifier in many different products. E465 and E466 are soluble, unlike the others.

Possible side effects Large concentrations of cellulose can cause problems in the intestine, ranging from diarrhoea to constipation.

E470 (i)-(iii)Fatty Acid Salts, E471 Mono- and Diglycerides of Fatty Acids, E472 Esters of Mono- and Diglycerides of Fatty Acids, E473 Sugar Esters of Fatty Acids, E474 Sucroglyceerides, E475 Polyclycerol Esters of Fatty Acid, E476 Polyglycerol Polyricinoleate, E477 Propane-1,2-diol Esters of Fatty Acids, E481 Sodium Stearoyl-2-lactylate, E482 Calcium Stearoyl-2-lactylate, E483 Stearyl Tartrate Made from mostly plant fats and used as emulsifiers and stabilisers in many products.

Possible side effects None known. A word of caution to certain religious groups and vegetarians: although mainly vegetable oils are used, animal fat (including pork) cannot be excluded.

E491 Sorbitane Mono Stearate, E492 Sorbitane Tri Stearate, E493 Sorbitane Mono Laurate, E494 Sorbitane Mono Oleate, E495 Sorbitane Mono Palmitate Made from a combination of sorbitol and stearic acid, a normal fatty acid from vegetable or animal origin, this is used as an emulsifier and stabiliser in a wide range of products.

Possible side effects None known. A word of caution to certain religious groups and vegetarians: although mainly vegetable oils are used, animal fat (including pork) cannot be excluded.

E500 (i)-(iii)Sodium Carbonates, E501 Potassium Carbonates, E501 Ammonium Carbonates, E504 Magnesium Carbonates Produced from seawater or salt, these are natural minerals used as acidity regulators and rising agents in many different products.
Possible side effects None known.

E507 Hydrochloric Acid A natural acid that is present in the stomach, produced from salt and sulphuric acid and used as an acidity regulator in cheese and beer.
Possible side effects None known.

E508 *Potassium Chloride* Natural salt used as a low-salt, low-sodium replacement.
Possible side effects None known.

E509 *Calcium Chloride* Natural salt used as an acidity regulator and to give firmness to fruit and vegetables.
Possible side effects None known.

E510 *Ammonium Chloride* Acidity regulator, flavouring and nutrient used in yeast-fermented products like bread.
Possible side effects None known.

E511 *Magnesium Chloride* Natural salt used to sterilise vegetables.
Possible side effects None known.

E512 *Stannous Chloride* Made from tin ores and hydrochloric acid and used as a stabiliser in tinned asparagus and beans.
Possible side effects None known.

E513 *Sulphuric Acid* Prepared from sulphur dioxide, oxygen and water and used as an acidity regulator in beer and cheese.
Possible side effects None known.

E514 *Sodium Sulphate* Made from salt and sulphuric acid, used in colourings and chewing gum as a filling agent and stabiliser.
Possible side effects None known.

E515 *Potassium Sulphate* Potassium salt and sulphuric acid mix used to treat water in brewing and as a salt replacement.
Possible side effects None known.

E516 *Calcium Sulphate* Prepared from calcium salts and sulphuric acid used as a firming agent and stabiliser, metal binding agent and nutrient in yeast for bread. Also in many pharmaceutical products.
Possible side effects None known.

E517 Ammonium Sulphate Used as a stabiliser in bakery and confectionery products, made up from ammonium salts and sulphuric acid.
Possible side effects None known.

E520 Aluminium Sulphate A natural mineral that is used as a clarification agent in the beer brewing process, it also strengthens the structure of vegetables during processing. Also used in pickled vegetables and to precipitate proteins as an anti-bacterial agent in deodorants.
Possible side effects None known.

E521 Aluminium-Sodium Sulphate An acidity regulator, strengthens vegetables in the processing stage and acts as a bleaching agent in flour. Also used in cheese and in confectionery.
Possible side effects None known.

E523 Aluminium-Ammonium Sulphate Stabiliser used in bakery products and colourings.
Possible side effects In high concentrations could inhibit absorption of vitamin B or threaten liver function.

E524 Sodium Hydroxide, E525 Potassium Hydroxide Strong alkali used as an acidity regulator and to enhance the industrial peeling of fruits, to blacken olives and in the preparation of caramel. In many products including baked goods, cocoa products, coffee creamer.
Possible side effects None known.

E526 Calcium Hydroxide, E 527 Ammonium Hydroxide An acidity regulator used in wine and also to preserve eggs. Mixed with sugar, it is also used to protect sweet frozen foods.
Possible side effects None known.

E528 Magnesium Hydroxide Used in cheese to enhance rennet, this strong alkali is used to regulate acidity, it is also used to preserve the colour of vegetables in the canning process.
Possible side effects Laxative effect in high concentrations.

E529 Calcium Hydroxide Made from chalk and used to treat intestines in sausage casings, also in bakery products.
Possible side effects None known.

E530 Magnesium Hydroxide, E535 Sodium Ferrocyanide, E536 Potassium Ferrocyanide, E538 Calcium Ferrocyanide Anti-caking agent used in cocoa and bakery products.
Possible side effects None known.

E541 Sodium Aluminium Phosphate Used as a raising agent in baking powder and in processed cheese.
Possible side effects Aluminium potentially impairs the calcium and phosphorous uptake by the body. The concentrations from E541 are generally so low that no effect is likely.

E551 Silicium Dioxide, E552 Calcium Silicate Used as an anti-caking agent to remove protein and yeast in beer and wine production and as an anti-foaming agent. Also used in many dry products.
Possible side effects None known.

E553 Magnesium Silicate, E554 Sodium Aluminium Silicate, E555 Aluminium Potassium Silicate, E556 Aluminium Calcium Silicate, E558 Bentonite An anti-caking and filling agent, also used as a coating, but mainly in cosmetics. E558 is also used as a clarifying agent in fruit juices.
Possible side effects None known.

E559 Aluminium Silicate (Kaolin) Fine, natural clay used as an anti-caking agent and carrier for aromas, it is found in instant coffee, milk powder and cosmetics and pharmaceutical preparations, mainly indigestion remedies.
Possible side effects None known.

E570 Stearic Acid Natural part of all fats and commercially produced from cottonseed oil, it is used as an anti-caking agent and plasticizer in chewing gum and flavourings but its main use is in cosmetics and pharmaceutical preparations.

Possible side effects None known. Although mainly extracted from plant sources, animal fat (including beef and pork) is sometimes used.

E574 Gluconic Acid, E575 Glucono-Delta-Lactone, E576 Sodium Gluconate, E577 Potassium Gluconate, E578 Calcium Gluconate, E579 Iron Gluconate A metal-binding agent that is either produced synthetically or produced by fungi from sugar. Used in fruit juices and jelly powder, instant puddings and custard powder. E578 is also used as a firming agent in processed vegetables.
Possible side effects None known.

E585 Ferrolactate Not, in fact, a milk-containing supplement, this is in fact an iron supplement added to infant milk formula.

E620 to E635 are all flavour enhancers, the most familiar of which is E621 Monosodium Glutamate (MSG) MSG has been accused of causing everything from cardiac disease to neurological dysfunction, including 'Chinese restaurant syndrome', (broncho-constriction in asthmatics), ADHD, autism, numbness, weakness, palpitations and aggression. Widely used in oriental cooking, especially Chinese food, where soy sauce is an essential ingredient. It is also found naturally in virtually all protein-containing foods. Monosodium glutamate is a salt of glutamic acid, one of the 20 amino acids that make up proteins. The human intestine has a voracious appetite for glutamate and uses up about 96 per cent of what we consume, so only perhaps 4 per cent remains in the body. As well as its natural sources, glutamate is added to soups, sauces, crisps, savoury and processed foods. Asian dishes that include soy or fish sauce use added glutamate as a flavour enhancer.
Possible side effects It is not necessary to separately detail all the flavour enhancers here, but a few specifics are worth noting: Asthmatics or anyone suffering from gout should avoid the guanylates and inosinates, E626 Guanylic acid, E627 Sodium guanylate, E628 Potassium guanylate, E629 Calcium guanylate, E630 Inosinic acid, E631 sodium inosinate, E632 Di-potassium

inosinate, E633 Calcium inosinate and E634 Calcium ribonu-cleotides.

Consumers are cautious about MSG and many are convinced that it is responsible for a range of health and wellbeing problems. Retailer advertising claiming 'no monosodium glutamate' has probably exacerbated that unease. However, double-blind, cross-over placebo-controlled studies have not confirmed any link.

The Joint Expert Committee on Food Additives of the United Nations (JECFA) placed MSG in the safest category of food additives. Later, both the Scientific Committee for Food of the United States (SCF) and the Federation of American Societies for Experimental Biology (FASEB) came to the same conclusion.

E640 Glycines A natural amino acid, a building block of protein, gylcine is mainly produced from gelatine, partly synthetic. It is used as a nutrient and flavour enhancer in bread.
Possible side effects None known. Glycine comes from gelatine, derived from animal bones, so it is not suitable for vegans or vegetarians.

E710 Spiramycins Spiramycins are a class of antibiotics, produced by the mould *Streptomyces ambofaciens*. They are used to inhibit the growth of fungi or mould in dairy, meat and egg products.
Possible side effects None known.

E713 Tylosin An antibiotic produced from the mould *Streptomyces fradiae*. Used to inhibit mould or fungi growth in dairy, meat and egg products.
Possible side effects None known.